MW01119897

'This is a very valuable and timely contribution to arts and mental health research and practice. Sagan provides a sensitive, thoughtful and nuanced consideration of this complex area, providing us with a very helpful overview of the debates surrounding arts, creativity and mental health. Her work is informed by wide scholarship, a careful awareness of her own position in the research and most importantly the stories of the artists with lived experience of mental ill health she has spoken to.'

– **Nick Rowe**, *PhD, Associate Professor,*
Director of Converge, York St John University, York, UK

'Sagan . . . unpacks and unpicks the gamut of previous research, writing, thinking and policy-making, as well as interrogating the criteria and language which under-pins it all. She also offers some findings from a large number of her interviews with people with lived experience, sometimes over many years. In her words, "These narratives also bring into question a commonly held belief that an analytic journey can only be undertaken through a professional intermediary."'

– **D Rosier**, *Artist, CEO of Experts by Experience, London, UK*

'Olivia Sagan's seminal book is a must read. In its scholarly research and eloquent, compassionate reflection and "organisation" of the narratives, it sheds necessary investigative light and contemporary discourse on the field of arts in health set against the historical landscape. It illuminates the nuances and complexities of the human story of mental illness and wellbeing putting at the forefront the individual's experience with creativity and visual arts.'

– **Helen Shearn**, *Head of Arts Strategy at South London*
and Maudsley NHS Foundation Trust, London, UK

Narratives of Art Practice and Mental Wellbeing

Narratives of Art Practice and Mental Wellbeing draws on extensive research carried out with mental health service users who are also practising artists. Using narrative data gained through hours of reflective conversation, it explores not whether art can contribute to positive wellbeing and improved mental health – as this is now established ground – but rather *how* art works, and the role art making can play in people's lives as they encounter crises, relapse, recovery or 'beyonding'.

The book maps the delicate ways in which finding a means to tell our story sometimes is the creative project we seek, and offers a reminder of how intrinsically linked our life trajectories are with creative opportunities. It describes the wide range of artistic activity occurring in health and community settings and the meanings of these practices to people with histories of mental turbulence. Drawing on psychoanalytic theory, the book explores the stories and various forms of visual arts practice spoken of, and considers the art-making processes, the creative moments and the objects which in some cases have changed people's lives.

The seven chapters of the book offer a blend of personal testimony, theory, debate, critique and celebration, and examine key topics of deliberation within the fields of art therapy, arts in health, community arts practice, participatory arts, and widening participation within arts education. It will be valuable reading for researchers, students, artists and practitioners in these fields.

Olivia Sagan is a Chartered Psychologist, Counsellor and Senior Lecturer in Psychology. She is currently Academic Co-ordinator for Psychology at Bishop Grosseteste University, Lincoln, UK.

Advances in Mental Health Research series

Books in this series:

The Clinical Effectiveness of Neurolinguistic Programming
A Critical Appraisal
Edited by Lisa Wake, Richard M. Gray & Frank S. Bourke

Group Therapy for Adults with Severe Mental Illness
Adapting the Tavistock Method
Diana Semmelhack, Larry Ende & Clive Hazell

Narratives of Art Practice and Mental Wellbeing
Reparation and connection
Olivia Sagan

Narratives of Art Practice and Mental Wellbeing

Reparation and connection

Olivia Sagan

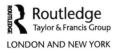

Routledge
Taylor & Francis Group

LONDON AND NEW YORK

First published 2015
by Routledge
27 Church Road, Hove, East Sussex, BN3 2FA

and by Routledge
711 Third Avenue, New York, NY 10017

Routledge is an imprint of the Taylor & Francis Group, an informa business

British Library Cataloguing in Publication Data
A catalogue record for this book is available from the British Library

Library of Congress Cataloging-in-Publication Data
Sagan, Olivia, author.
  Narratives of art practice and mental wellbeing : reparation and
  connection / Olivia Sagan.
      p. ; cm.
    Includes bibliographical references.
  I. Title. [DNLM: 1. Art Therapy. 2. Mental Disorders--therapy. 3. Art.
  4. Creativity. 5. Mental Health Services. WM 450.5.A8]
  RC489.A7
  616.89′1656–dc23   2014018714

ISBN: 978-0-415-82112-4 (hbk)
ISBN: 978-0-203-56904-7 (ebk)

Typeset in Baskerville
by Keystroke, Station Road, Codsall, Wolverhampton

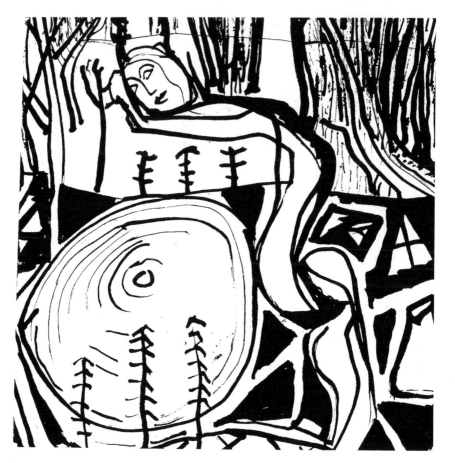

Inner journey

στην λεονορα, η κορη μου, για τα φτερα σου

Моєму батькові, за історії, які він ніколи мені не розказав

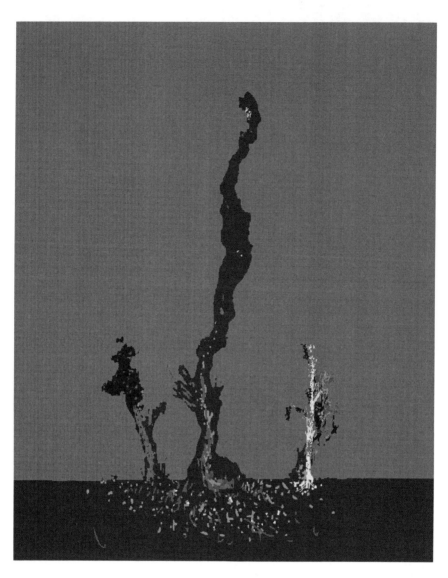

Charcoal woman

Contents

Illustrations

The copyrights of the images below remain with the artists.

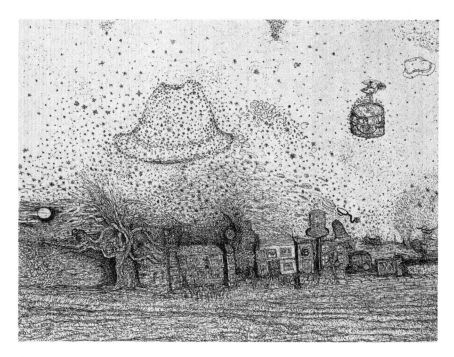

Cosmic hat

Foreword

Olivia Sagan has spent a great deal of time in conversation, or interview, with artists who have been, or are, subject to the attentions of the mental health system, the psychotherapies and institutionalized psychiatry. It matters not to her whether they regard themselves as professionals or outsiders, whether the art comes out of love, rage or quest, or whether they make it for work, therapy or leisure. At the heart of her inquiry is the relationship between creativity, identity and the capacity for connection, and as such she has much to tell us about a wider human impulse to make art.

This is a book that foregrounds the voices – and the suffering – of the people who told her their stories and shared their thoughts. These voices do not so much illustrate as deliver the argument. However, Sagan's scholarship also beams through. Her plurivocal work speaks to a subject of fascination and controversy – the connection between art and madness and how it has been presumed or disputed from Greek philosophy through the origins of psychiatry to contemporary neuropsychology. Sagan charts this history for us with cautious discrimination asking why we should have found this link so tantalizing, across disciplines, cultures and histories. Then, leaving the question open she turns to the experiences of the artists she has interviewed foregrounding their words, while interweaving them with her own analysis. She brings to the subject a distinctive perspective of post-Freudian object relations theory, and contextualizes it within the contemporary politics of art and health.

She sets out to add to the burgeoning art and mental health literature, not so much another study on the efficacy of art from a health perspective, as an attempt to understand how it does what it does for its makers. What she delivers, in a still undertheorized field, is a discussion that is historically framed, empirically grounded and theoretically elaborated from a perspective that extends beyond the therapeutic into aesthetic and emotional experience. The experience in question is that of 'ordinary' art making, albeit by people who are sometimes in 'extra-ordinary' states of mind. As such it illuminates the connection between mind and art well beyond the fields of mental illness, therapy or recovery.

This is of course uncertain territory in which the voices she records reveal that art can be used for expression or ejection of destructiveness and misery as much as for hope and repair. It is a welcome corrective to the impression given at times by arts and health advocates – for understandable political reasons – that art is unproblematically beneficent in health care, and that it simply remains for the evidence base to accumulate, and policy makers to take note. This book has an altogether grittier texture which sits uneasily with those aspects of the recovery movement drawn to positive psychology and happiness science. Speaking, as they do, from 'wellness' and the non-pathologized parts of the self can serve to support hope and resist stigmatization, but the discourse of recovery is strongly normative at times, and can itself take on the aspect of an ideology. The responsibility to recover and be well may be experienced by some as an empowering spur to self-efficacy, but the suffering of those who fail will be stamped with desolation and futility. If the generalization of recovery discourse develops in the absence of a range of mental health resources that offer an individuated approach, including those which allow for the full expression of disturbance and despair, the recovery movement unwittingly aligns with the neo-liberalization of health care. In such a model the withdrawal of public provision demands of individuals an increasing ability to look after themselves and a reconstruction of health-care subject as utility-maximizing rational chooser, 're-tooled' for productivity in the workplace. It pre-supposes a health-care system in which there is little patience and even affordability for the expression of existential crisis and its working through. The re-symboliza-tion of relationship between mind, body and world that art making allows is beyond its scope. Under these conditions arts provision will gain the support of health professionals and policy makers to the extent that it offers a cost-effective route to self-responsibility. However, this is an arena in which people in the mental health system have 'failed' by definition.

Rational choice theory has nothing to tell us of the artists who speak through this book. If there is one point that emerges more strongly than any other it is that they make art to deal with overwhelming anxiety and with the irreconcilable conflicts and paradoxes of existence. They project into their art the shards of the self and they use it not so much to unite the fragments as to hold, contain or bind them into a symbolic form. It is a work of repair forever in progress and forever vulnerable to disintegration. The voices recorded by Sagan remind us that individuals may frame their illness narratives as 'quest', but rather than any simple quest for 'recovery', or even for meaning, this may be a quest for the kind of psychosocial integration that allows for a bearable co-existence with one's demons. It may be even here that creativity resides.

Sagan cautions us against the romanticization of suffering while according the misery of madness its own dignity: the voices in her book render it intelligible through their own accounts of their need to make art. Alongside these voices she brings to bear a secular theoretical perspective which can do justice not only to the existence of mental suffering but to its experience. Object relations theory offers an account of the dissolution of a coherent sense of self; of the impulsion to evacuate the fragments; and of their potential for re-integration through the forms and figures of art. What this book adds is the firsthand account of artists who have undergone – are still undergoing – those processes. And that experience becomes recognizable to the reader insofar as disowning distress and rage, and expelling it into people and objects, is a 'normal madness' in which we can all at times partake. What keeps that madness manageable for most of us, most of the time, is the re-introjection of the experience of its containment – through other people and the cultural forms of everyday life. There is more work to be done here in understanding how it is that when the functional aesthetics of everyday experience disintegrates we are left with a feeling that Bion so evocatively termed 'nameless dread'. Sagan's interviewees do give us glimpses of this, but the fact that they can talk of it means that the dread, if not named, has already been drawn, painted, carved, moulded or woven through their art.

What the interviews reveal to us is something of how the artists 'work with' their art as well as 'working through', and how this happens both within and without the formal therapeutic contexts of art therapy. Indeed this is not primarily a book about art therapy (though it will be of interest to the art therapeutic community) but about how people develop resilience by making artwork for themselves and others. As such it has much to say about the subjective struggle of artists with their material. The voices within it are irreducibly individual while at the same time, for the main part, seeking connection with a human community.

If the reader is looking for yet more support for art making's contribution to positive mental health outcomes, they will find it in some measure, but Sagan presents a complex view, and this makes it not so much a cheerleader as a nuanced addition to the arts and health field. Its power lies in the interweaving of voice and theory – always a difficult accomplishment – achieved here with fluency and verve. What we have is an account of the place of art making in a narrative quest for a tolerably, though always imperfectly, integrated self able to connect with a wider world of other selves; and of the place of art making and the art object as the point around which this endeavour revolves.

> Art making, and the other it imagines, or to which it relates in the group, thus may offer opportunities for a social mending; between one's self and others, and between one and a group, between groups and other groups, through a focus centred on the art object – and its making, or coming to be. Some artists felt this touched on what it was to be human.

Lynn Froggett
Professor of Psychosocial Welfare
University of Central Lancashire, UK

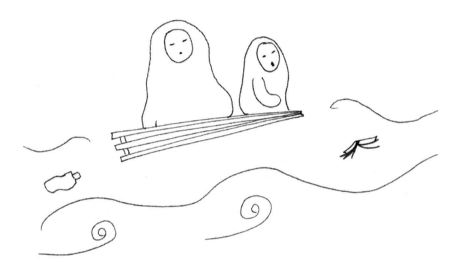

We're adrift

Acknowledgements

There are a great many people who are owed a debt of gratitude for their part in the writing of this book. First and foremost, my thanks go to the many artists who agreed to be interviewed and gave so generously of their stories. My thanks also go to individuals who have been participants, collaborators, data collectors, film and image makers, transcribers and general supporters of any one of the projects that have led to this book.

Colleagues Helen Shearn, Maxine Walker, Emily Candela and Mark Crawley must also receive thanks for their support of this book and, more importantly, their work advocating the arts in the lives of people with mental health difficulties. Colleagues Emily Candela, Sue Hacking, Antigonos Sochos and Angie Voela who have offered important critical readings of first drafts of this book, are thanked heartily for their diligent suggestions. Errors and weaknesses that remain are my fault entirely.

The Arts Council England, the University of the Arts London, South London & Maudsley Charitable Trust and Bishop Grosseteste University Lincoln are all thanked too, for their financial support.

I would like to give thanks and acknowledge the artists whose images appear in this book. Their contributions do what images do best – make words seem somewhat superfluous.

And finally, as ever, my thanks, gratitude and love to my partner and family who are ever supportive of my need to be quiet and be alone.

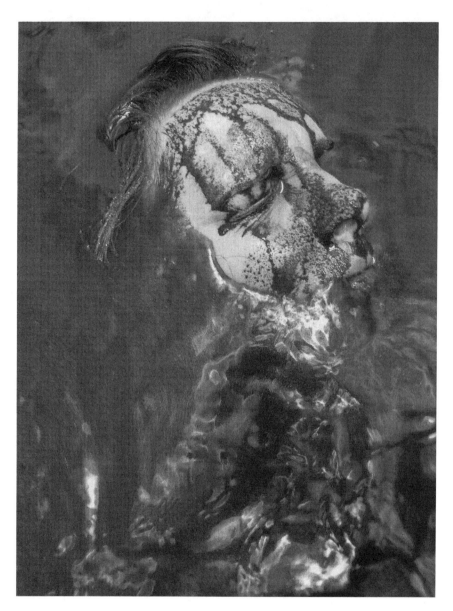

Curdled self portrait 2014

1 Chris, Kandinsky and the autobiography of the question

A brief introduction

Chris comes into the small white room. The security guard accompanying him catches my eye, gives me a short nod and leaves us. Chris makes the briefest of eye contact, and then carefully sets down a rolled-up poster. I quietly ask after him as I unpack his paints and lay out a few basic tools including a plastic cup of water. Chris is, as ever, very quiet, gentle and slow in his responses. An ethereal looking man of about 25, he gives the impression of being younger – and of having left, or leaving, or never having quite arrived.

He unrolls his poster: Kandinsky's Squares with Concentric Circles. I unroll the watercolour copy that he has been working on with me, for weeks. He sets to work, eagerly, hungrily; mixing colours, looking quickly from poster to copy to paints. Now and then he shoots me a look, and I see his eyes are bright, animated; there is colour to his face, and his features are held in concentration, an expression of intensity yet relaxation, of arrival. He feels more in the room now.

I don't know how the painting is working on him, in him – either the original or the copy, or the process of bringing the two into some imagined alignment. But for a short session, week after week, something important is happening for Chris. And for me too.

With this encounter some years ago in a high security psychiatric ward, I began my wondering at the frisson of art meeting the troubled mind and its sadnesses. Not long afterwards I began the research path that led to the narratives in this book. And as any presentation of the stories of others should start with who the listener is, allow me in this introductory chapter a brief autobiographical note.

Such an autobiographic note is perhaps overdue. In researching this book I was often taken aback by the generosity and openness of people who shared their stories while often knowing so little about me. But one day, after speaking briefly with a man who had decided not to consent to an interview, I realized that his understandable assumptions about me were born of my approach to this research. This has been to foreground others as much as possible, and keep the reflexive, autobiographic side of this endeavour to myself – appearing, no doubt, aloof at times, and less generous with my story than people were with theirs. There were conflicting positionings in this research, each of which had its own forcefield that attracted and repelled the other at different moments. One position issued from my work as researcher in which a certain amount of self-disclosure is acceptable – even desirable depending on your approach; while another came from my work as counsellor, where it is rarely helpful or acceptable in the clinical relationship for the counsellor story, in whatever distilled form, to be shared. So I offer here, in this introductory space to the chapters that follow, some background to the auto-biography of the question which lay behind the interviews in this book – *what is the experience of art practice in the lives of people with histories of mental ill health.*

My fascination for voice, narrative and creative ways of building a life story is rooted in my own family history, in watching people close to me struggle for, and with, words. Early on in my life it became clear to me that stories both soothed trouble and caused trouble – and yet they always battled to be told, a telling whose contested nature I describe in Chapter 4 of this book. This early home-front history would steer me at first, precariously, into the visual arts (Sagan, 2007a) and arts applications, where I became aware maybe for the first time of two persisting fundamentals. One, that class and its bestowed privilege and haphazardly allo-cated lack not only regulates one's access to mainstream culture but dominates it; and two, in the collateral damage of the British class system there are stifled lives yet incredible, ignited stories. These stories, of how individuals get caught up, pulled along and sometimes pulled under by poverty, illness and distress, talked to me not only of the rough tides of these lives, but of the ingenious ways that people found to navigate them.

Later, once I began teaching in community learning organizations, with their draughty, one-bar-electric-fire, mugs-of-tea settings, I was struck again by the stories of resourcefulness and resilience, particularly amongst learners for whom the very business of learning was fraught, and the enterprise of daily life no less so. My years as a teacher of adult learners were also busy with opportunities for me to observe the impact of learning and art making in the lives of institutionalized mental health patients, some of whom, like Chris, I grew to know over a sustained period of time. My vignette at the beginning of this chapter is from notes I made while teaching in a high security psychiatric hospital – a rare experience rich in moments of wonder, confusion and dismay.

In working daily with this array of learners, the mentally ill, the refugee, the homeless, the battered and the isolated, I was struck by how, in the words of Nobel Prize winner Rabindranth Tagore (2002), 'Thought feeds itself with its own words and grows'. I watched and listened as learning, in these relatively safe spaces, seemed to embellish people's stories with more subtle words, a deeper access to their personal biographies and sometimes a greater range of choices about who they could become. In both art and pedagogy, I began feeling my way along the contours of the tricky and delicate interface of learning, creativity and mental illness (Sagan, 2012), and so began a fascination for the numerous struggles I saw people grapple with, and the often complex strategies they developed in order to live better lives.

On later becoming a counsellor, the story listener *par excellence*, in hindsight an almost inevitable move, the intrigue continued, now for the way in which stories in the therapeutic setting, no less an educational space, appeared to frame, limit or even release people. I eventually began to 'do research' – what the wonderful anthropologist and novelist Zora Neale Hurston (1891–1960) called 'formalized curiosity'. First this formalized curiosity led me to look at the written words of those with histories of mental illness, then to looking at their art work, and to what their stories told me about their encounter with each. A short time later my father, who for decades had suffered a shifting and perplexing mental illness, died (Sagan, 2013), but not before showing me again what I had found repeatedly in my research – that the story we construct and the life that we remember *demand* expression. This story is re-made and its telling rendered even more mysterious by age, and, in my father's case, by Alzheimer's. Observing my father's final struggle with the disease, in a life full of literal war, personal battles, attacks both real and imagined followed by their copious and necessary defences, I was to be reminded once again how fragile yet durable and always extraordinary the human mind is. Theory, whichever – take your pick – by which to understand it, can only barely scratch the surface.

The fascination for this listening to stories of lives has never left me. It returns to me now as I listen to the interviews for this book again. And in working with the transcripts or listening to the pauses and chuckles and sobs and silences – brought into play once more is a long-term and ambivalent relationship with stories. This ambivalence warns me that stories are fickle – the speaker and the seduced listener are performing an intricate inter-subjective dance which is co-constructed within the bounds of this particular moment and relationship; and yes, stories are slippery – the very words we speak are full of the voices of others and the multifarious tricks of memory and connection. In Riessman's words, 'The "truths" of narrative accounts lie not in their faithful representation of a past world, but in the shifting connections they forge between past, present, and future' (2002: 705). In Chapters 4, 5 and 6, I try to trace these connections between a story's past, present and future, and look at the role of art, in helping make, identify and question such connections. So this book is born of my fascination; for story, for art making, for health – and the curious ways in which these are interlinked.

In every story there is a nugget that emerges as the teller weaves her story of past, present and future. A nugget not of 'truth' or of the essential being of the teller, but a nugget of *sense*, for want of a better word, a resonant something that leads us to think otherwise about the story, about the experience, about the teller, and, if we use our antennae, about the listener. That nugget can be taken and worked with, as I have tried to do across this research. Magpie-like, I have descended on these stories and tried to get hold of how art works for people when pretty much all else fails. And that's what this book offers. Organized nuggets. Organized through the filter of me and turned over in my hands while shining a soft light on each one, a light of theories and observations which have been shown, for me, to light a way to some better excavation.

So who are you, reading this book? Such organized nuggets may interest you if, like me, like so many of the people in this book, you have questions about the relationship between what we think, how we feel and what we do. These questions are the bedrock of both psychology and philosophy, but I offer rather less elevated, working examples of this relationship, drawn from the experiences of the people with whom I spoke. You may be an artist yourself. You may be at an early stage of wondering about the relationship between who you are and the work you produce – in which case the book will offer an introduction to a rich literature connecting the unconscious, with its strata of memory, fears, joys and yearning, to our creative outputs. You may be a student in the area of mental health, planning to become a counsellor perhaps, or a community health professional. You may have already come across the use of First Person Narratives through the work, for example, of Gail Hornstein in the US. It has impressed you, perhaps, as a means by which to understand better and more respectfully the people with whom you may already be working; people for whom mental illness and its DSM 5 diagnoses are stuck like limpets across their case notes, whilst they simultaneously live lives which are complex, often difficult, and sometimes ingeniously creative.

Or you may yourself be just such a person. Tired, perhaps, of the sedimented, medical version of who you are. Troubled by that version, one that prescribes what your 'condition' and therapeutic regime are and what they limit you to. Perhaps you are busy with managing your own life strategies and have an inkling that making art helps forge another version of yourself – by chiselling a life story through alternative means of working with your past and its cicatrices, your breakthroughs and your beyond. To you then, a special welcome is extended. For after years of listening to the stories of mental health service users; survivors; the mentally ill; the mad; however you have positioned yourselves before me and my recording device, I do know that your stories about your experiences don't 'just' tell us about you – they tell us about us; the 'sane' – and our frightfully sane society.

You may have opened this book because its title pinged onto one of your devices and you are one of a growing number of artists who, for your own multifaceted reasons, are working in an 'Arts in Health' context, and have long been asking some of the questions alighted on in this book. Questions such as those in Chapter 3, perhaps, about where and how your art practice and its applications touch or have touched the lives of people with mental health difficulties. In that case Chapter 3 may be of special interest to you, where people describe their artful encounters and transitions as they moved in work and identity from, in some instances, easel in a psychiatric ward to one-person exhibitions in the world outside the psychiatric cloister.

Perhaps you are a psychologist or researcher working in the expanding field of narrative psychology – exploring the mysteries and few certainties regarding the interplay between who we are, how we become so, how we tell that story and what impact on our wellbeing that telling and disclosure has. A study whose interplay was the stuff of Freud's cases as he scrutinized the stories of people in distress and what their unguarded and free-associative words might reveal about the genesis of that distress and its particular ways of telling itself. Psychology, in getting over its long-standing anxiety about both qualitative research and the legacy of narrative being traced back to psychoanalytic interest in the spoken word, is readier now, to include narrative into its disciplinary fold, and steadier too, its relationship with stories of mental illness and how they inform psychological knowledge.

You may, finally, be researching the impact of arts on the lives of people outside the mainstream; the impact of arts participation and the means by which people access arts activity. You could well be part of a growing body of people who, aware of the mounting evidence of a correlative or even causative link between art and wellbeing, are wishing to explore what people say about this link and in some way evaluate the impact of art in their lives. Or maybe you are none of these readers. Perhaps you have picked this book up on a bench in a train station in line with one of those serendipitous laws that dictate that we come across the books we need to. Maybe before the train arrives you will be inspired by the narratives in this book to ask the questions: am I living my life as creatively, as congruently, as I can? How do I choose to tell my story?

You may be all or some of the above, depending on the day, your role and your hat. Indeed, in my talking to people about arts activity and mental health, I often tripped up on their roles, my assumptions and the play of disciplinary languages in whose cross-purpose interactions misunderstandings sometimes run rampant. People who were community artists mentioned a history of depression, of break-down, or, in a throwaway line, the fact that they 'started painting after their first suicide attempt'. Their 'research' was their art and their illness; their 'practice' both their art and their mental health work in the community. People I engaged with in their role as project workers, busily organising budgets and venues, turned out to be service users or part-time lecturers in Fine Art. People I thought were art students turned out to be – as well as art students – residents of therapeutic communities and community activists . . . and people who I thought were mental health service users were . . . service users, but also, it turned out, sometimes managed high-profile arts projects, or had done research into schizophrenia and symbolism; ran successful companies, painted gorgeous landscapes, wrote, ran marathons, climbed mountains. You get the picture – and it is a picture familiar to anyone who has stepped into mental health settings for any short period of time. It is also not new to anyone who has stepped into *life* for any short period of time, as the first thing to be learned is that people are, and are not, what we think they are; they, we, are always so much more.

So how can this book be read? Well, it can be dipped in to, glanced at, picked up and put down, or read cover to cover. As I tell my students, however, the latter should only be attempted with any non-fiction book for very good reasons known only to the reader. You may, in either case, want to pause to enjoy the images, question them, wonder at them. I suspect the best way to read the book is by first looking at parts that resonate with your own area of experience or interest. You will find that chapters vary in how many references are included and how much theory they contain. Some chapters, for example Chapter 2, where I give a historical foothold in the area of research into mental illness and creativity, are reference-heavy; others, where I include theory I have found useful in trying to understand some of the mental processes involved in making art and how these aid wellbeing, for example Chapters 5 and 6, are more theory-heavy. In both cases I hope that the references and theory I have chosen to include point the reader usefully in a solid direction for further investigation – rather than serve to cloud and deter from the experiences of people, and the questions such experiences raise. There is a wealth of material now in the area of art and mental health, and I hope you, the reader, will be inspired to explore it further if you have not already begun to do so.

This formalized curiosity

My research background roots its ethical stance and approach in the feminist research paradigm that spoke loudly of collaboration; of participation, and of 'giving voice'. Of course, the road is muddied and bloodied now – collaboration and participation are questioned with more acuity today in terms of power and critiqued more finely in terms of access and asymmetry – areas of unrest of which I offer more detail in Chapter 3. Collaboration is now increasingly online, with virtual relationships usurping those in the flesh, and international, global forums are possible in a way that only small local groupings were possible in the past. It is potentially just as easy for someone in the UK to collaborate with a peer in Arcadia, Arizona as one in Litherland, Liverpool. In terms of voice, the internet and its now myriad social networking opportunities is potentially better at 'giving' this than researchers, and voice itself is more heavily contested, as is the 'truth' of the words which we speak – a point to which I return in Chapter 4. In tandem is the challenge of working with the 'self' in what Bauman (2000) referred to as 'liquid modernity', wherein we are all more changeable and open to multiple (re-)creations than ever before. A change of autobiography is as simple as a change of avatar. In these Facebooked days, with the multiple potentialities for reconfigurations and perhaps multiple errors of memory and history, we are just as likely to be worried about the right to be forgotten as we are the right to be heard. Many of these challenges prompt us to hold in mind that we are in a research era where questions about how 'new' knowledge is formulated, disseminated, used and by whom – are more pressing than ever.

The tense, messy, unpredictable and shifting character of the research in which many qualitative researchers are involved tells us something straight off the bat about investigations into human experience. This message – that human experience is itself tense, messy, unpredictable and shifting – is one which quantitative research does not address, cleansed as it is of such human features and focused as it is on other questions and ways of measuring their answers. Qualitative research, at its best, takes as its very material the 'unclear'. The 'surplus' that is so irksome to positivistic research and the very notion of the 'outlier' – become the very core of our endeavour. In choosing not only to not omit the unclear and the outlier, but instead to work with them, we endeavour to avoid the pitfall described by German theoretical physicist Werner Heisenberg who suggested that when research omits all that is unclear, we are left with 'completely uninteresting and trivial tautologies' (Heisenberg, 1971: 213).

Mike White (2005) amongst others argues that testimony from people is increasingly regarded as a valid form of 'evidence' despite the continued clarion call to positivistic means by which to count, measure and offer statistically significant proofs of X. Such a turn in the face of the still dominant trend, gradual as it is, is indicative of an ongoing dissatisfaction with an understanding of the world based in what French philosopher Auguste Comte (1853) saw as the 'Third Phase' of the human intellectual process. Viewing these phases, which journey from the theological through the metaphysical and into the scientific way of understanding nature and the social world, helps us to locate the current 'medicalization' of mental illness, and the pull towards positivist means by which to explore and measure it. A mature third stage sees us questioning more ardently than ever what particular baby we have thrown out with the proverbial bathwater of the previous two stages and what we can reshape and refine with our twenty-first-century sensibilities. And this is the task for qualitative research as it explores the changing face, nature and experience of mental ill health. The positivists have a simple solution: the world must be divided into that which we can say clearly and the rest, which we had better pass over in silence. But surely, if we omitted all that is unclear we would indeed be left with completely uninteresting and trivial tautologies. The now even wider and more sensitive range of qualitative methods includes 'important tools for a deeper evaluation of arts-based interventions' (Clift, 2012: 123). The researchers of what are increasingly referred to as 'complex interventions' – interventions in health care which have multiple components – must draw on and develop every tool in the box to delve into the experience being investigated, and that of the researchers undertaking the investigation (Froggett and Hollway, 2010). So this book, far from being a call to disregard quantitative methods of investigating how art impacts on our lives and wellbeing, hopes to be a reminder of how subtle that impact is, and how careful our listening needs to be in its role as research tool.

These postmodern research themes and the ontological anxiety that inevitably accompanies such epistemological rug-pulling now need to be framed by post-boom austerity and two major questions to emerge from the dust. One asks us to look afresh at ethical conduct in all institutional processes and the politics of concealment, accountability and transparency. While governments struggle to keep a lid on a rash of leaks and whistleblowing activity and difficult questions are being asked about the tension between the right to know and the need to conceal, some of the older questions which lurk behind issues raised in this book, about diagnosis, the right to self-determine and how we care for our citizens, are being surveyed afresh. Another interlinked question with a presence in this book asks what we mean by happiness and wellbeing, now that it is clearer than ever that there is no correlation between these, the climate of capitalism with the gloves off and our frenzied accumulation of material wealth. These two pressing items on the post-developed nations' agenda have triggered moves towards greater collaboration, both macro and micro; and a new attention given to the power and potential of multidisciplinarity as a means by which to generate less myopic approaches and more creative solutions – both of which are pressing needs when looking to support mental health and wellbeing in an economically constrained, cold climate.

So what of the small picture in all this – the story of this particular piece of formalized curiosity? It began, as mentioned, with Chris and Kandinsky. It took further shape as I interviewed and observed a group of long-term mental health service users on a longitudinal project (Sagan, 2007b) and began to trust in the inherent usefulness to the interviewee of the interviews themselves and the ways of knowing that I felt leaked into the exchanged words and the silences that punctuated them. There was a turning point in this work as an interviewer which gave me further insight into the ways in which life, story and understanding are melded. It was to colour my research thereafter and so is one which I will briefly relate.

Marge, a 'service user' in her late sixties who lived with physical ill health, a disability and Obsessive Compulsive Disorder, was a woman of few words – or as her case notes had it, 'low verbal ability'. She agreed, nevertheless, to a series of interviews with me to tell me about her life. Here is a vignette from my notes at the time:

> *As Marge sits down, her walking stick, which she has leant carefully on the chair before taking her seat, slides down onto the floor with a clatter. She casts me a fleeting glance, smiles nervously and gets up to retrieve it. She slowly leans the stick again on exactly the same spot, and struggles to control her hand which continues its customary shaking. Lowering her painful bulk into the chair again, the stick once more slides to the floor. Marge looks at me again and again rises, with more tired difficulty to retrieve it. This is repeated four or five times with growing tension before Marge finally, exhausted and defeated, lays the stick lengthways on the floor. She continues to shoot it sidelong, disturbed glances for the next half hour. We both know it is not in the 'right' place. It has become the story of the interview.*

> *And there it is; there it is. One of those intense, short-lived immersions into a private, everyday battle: with a walking stick that won't be still; with age and infirmity; with the repetitive demands of compulsion. And there it is too, the suspension in a borderland – as I sit, fascinated and appalled at my observing and not doing in this intimacy, suspended in inactivity between the possible doing of being human and the observing impotence of the researcher's gaze. It is a tight moment in which Marge gifts me with a cameo of her life and both lives her story through its telling and tells it through its living.*

Marge showed me it is important to not only hear the stories in the interviews but to see them, and also reminded me how discomfort and even pain will be endured by people who feel the call to tell it. Interviews, given and taken in a facilitating and sensitive way, seemed to offer an opportunity for the teller not simply to repeat but to reconfigure; to play with emerging meanings and to take stock, revaluate and literally *re-count*. Marge later made a gentle joke in her broad Yorkshire accent about our 'stick interview' as she called it, and while brushing it off lightly made reference to the fact that '. . . *you would have waited all day, love, I weren't used to that . . .*'.

I was influenced too, in my researcher journey, by both Wengraf (2001) and Hollway and Jefferson (2000) and to this day hold that the biographic narrative interview offers a unique way into thick data of ontological depth which can offer a glimpse of meaning making in people's lives. I soon began a longer-term project; to interview people who had histories of mental ill health who were visual art makers.

Continuing to adhere to a psychosocial model of the person, recognizing that both social influences and psychological forces work on the ways in which we shape and tell our life, I drew on phenomenological approaches in research to work with the narratives, looking to stay close to the 'nub' of the experience being described, talking to people, listening to them carefully, staying curious and open to surprise – and keeping their stories alive for what they elucidate about illness, art making, resilience and social barriers. There was a to-ing and fro-ing, an iterative some-times cyclical movement, between myself, the narrators and the phenomenon being described – in the non-linear and immersive nature of phenomenological research:

> Whatever variant of phenomenology, the task remains profoundly dialectical: researchers need to straddle subjectivity and objectivity, intimacy and distance, being inside and outside, being a part of and a part from, bracketing the self and being self-aware . . .
>
> (Finlay, 2014: 124)

The research took me again to questions of ethics, reflexivity and being – in particular being open. As Dahlberg and colleagues (2008: 98) describe in their phenomenological approach to reflective lifeworld research, openness is the very 'mark' of a willingness to understand. Such openness involves, they urge, 'respect and a certain humility toward the phenomenon, as well as sensitivity and flexi-bility'. For this book, I engaged in interviews with more than sixty people each of whom summoned in some way my ability, weakness or authenticity with regard to the question: what are the constituent elements of openness, respect and humility in research? The question is alive to me now, and its aliveness, rather than its answer, is what remains important.

So what of these people who perhaps unknowingly pushed me on a bit in my understandings – how do they appear, or sometimes not appear, in this book? Who are these artists who were so open with their disclosures? The participants whose narratives are extracted in this book had varying degrees of contact with me and the research. Some were instrumental in the research design of different projects, or took part in some of the photographing and filming in those projects, or joined discussions about the scope and destination of the research. I have had contact with a small number of these people over a period of years and have been able to watch their practice grow. A beautiful print arrived in the post not long after I began this book from one woman artist who I haven't seen in person for years but who has kept in light touch. It simply delighted me – not only as a piece of art but because of the stories it brought back through its colours – stories of the ways in which she lived her life, faced her illness and worked her art. Curiously, as this book was being edited I dreamt that my house was burgled and this print was the only thing stolen. Make of that what you will – I have my own hunches; about receiving, about losing, and the parts of self which may be felt impervious or vulnerable to each.

Other participants I have spoken to only once – or, in a very small number of cases, in line with their preference for no spoken contact, people have emailed me their thoughts and reflections regarding their art practice and their well-being. In each case what was crucial was that the person whose story was being given remained comfortable with the process; that informed consent was given (Faulkner, 2004) and that the level of contact between us was felt to be non-intrusive and respectful. I am privileged to have worked with each person, seen her work and heard his stories.

Confidentiality is always a far more complex issue than is routinely portrayed by the literature on research. Each participant in this book has agreed to varying levels of exposure and this book makes use of both people's real names and pseudonyms, respectively, as requested. A few participants who wished for greater levels of anonymity asked that certain details of their lives not be revealed, or other details be deliberately changed. In one or two cases individuals revised their consent for me to use specific parts of their interview as publication drew near, in response to family requests or changes in life circumstances that made the original testimony and exposure more risky or potentially unsettling. I hope I have been sufficiently sensitive and accommodating to these varied requests. Recognition via association with another participant is always a slim possibility in some cases, but I have endeavoured, where people have requested maximum confidentiality, to ensure that their identities and connections with others are obscured.

Yet multiple factors made my research slip through my fingers – interviews in a small number of cases, for one user-led project in particular, were filmed and the audio-visual clips sometimes requested by the participant, after which point they had the right to do with these as they pleased including placing them on their own or others' websites. Some people also had their own websites with catalogued work which they were happy for me to look at and refer to – which immediately fuzzied the levels of confidentiality I could offer if I were to link them to these sites. Some artists referred to exhibitions in their stories that again could, through association, reveal their identity if the information was not obscured. Such questions about anonymity, confidentiality and the extent to which licence was given for stories to be altered to protect these endured. The border between public and private was continually challenged, with seepage through image, voice, dissemination, disclosure. The shifts of visibility and invisibility, of disclosing and displaying, proved a research challenge but also a fascinating entry into the ways in which art itself can function in the lives of those for whom invisibility and disclosure are potent terms, a theme explored in Chapter 6.

The people I spoke with ranged in age from 19 to 67, were predominantly White British, although there are also people from Black African, Indian Asian, European, American, Russian and South East Asian backgrounds. This book does not endeavour to explore cultural influences on how art was used by them – nor does it make comment on how gender, age or dis/ability enters the narratives, although all these are pressing avenues for investigation of the ways in which identity is sought; forged; lost and found. The majority of the participants came from lower socioeconomic backgrounds – although this status was complicated by the mobility (usually downwards) which people experience as a result of continuing mental ill health and the barriers and stigma strewn across any paths towards employment, career progression, economic stability. What all participants have in common is a history of mental ill health, a formal diagnosis and a passion for making art. Each easily identified with calls made through mental health and art networks and word of mouth in the South East of Britain for people to talk to me about their experiences in these areas. In terms of their art practice, the only stipulation I made for the interviewees was that they be involved in the making of visual art. There were people who contacted me from the performing arts and even more who were involved in creative writing – but they have not been interviewed or kept in the 'sample'.

All interviews were digitally recorded with the consent of the interviewee. In some cases more than one interview was conducted with the participant; and the interviews lasted between twenty minutes and almost two hours. On some occasions the interviewee emailed me later, to say s/he had something to add, or to request that we speak again. In each case, my priority was ensuring the participant felt that she/he had told me as much or as little of their story as they wished, rather than seeking an adherence to a particular methodological design. The interviews were typically unstructured, with an open invitation for people to tell me the story of their life. In some cases no further questions were asked. In others, people requested that I be more specific, and guide them towards areas that I wanted them to tell me about. In these cases the questions were open, covering three areas: one's life story; mental health difficulties experienced; and one's art practice. Typically these questions were: 'tell me about your life'; 'can you say more about your health problems' and 'how would you describe your art practice?' Frequently, and fruitfully, I simply said: 'tell me more about that'.

All the interviews I did were transcribed verbatim, and, in line with the original research design, loaded onto NVivo software which allows for an analysis of, amongst other things, emerging themes. For this book, however, it became important to go back to the sound files themselves, listening and re-listening to all the interviews, in, what a colleague of mine once described as, a 'cozying up to the data'. There were reasons for this. I had a strong sense that software restrictions (including its appearance, assumptions and language) placed a distance between me, the listener or reader and the type of experience being described (Langdridge, 2007). It is all too easy in research for the methodology to get in the way of the people; and for processes, be they analysis, dissemination, writing a paper or, in this case, a book, to become the primary, rather than secondary task. Going back to actually hearing people's pauses, sobs, laughter, stutters and elegant or clumsy turns of phrase brought back the experience that was being looked at, immediately – sometimes with a new apprehending of possible meaning. Every time I lost track of the task, or became overwhelmed by the demands of compiling and writing a book, or lost faith in my ability to do justice to the interviews – I would go back, to the stories, to the sound files, to the people, in as whole a form as I had; not to the transcriptions or the software. These seemed to further disembody the participants, to condense them into themes, to collapse their free associations into less free dissociations. As I mention in Chapter 5, one thing mentioned by very many participants was a loathing of categorization and the ways in which they had as artists and as mental health service users been defined by systems, words, diagnoses and imposed boundaries of what might be possible.

Indeed one of my misgivings in presenting the narratives in the way that I have in this book is that inevitably, the depth, idiosyncrasy and richness of the *person* are lost. This may be because of the processes of selection and extraction, because the 'person' is not presented with all of her biographical details (usually at the wish of the speaker), but also because of a rather more enigmatic variable, that of language itself, and its limits in describing experiences beyond reason, such as mental illness. Jacques Derrida (2005: 65) maintained that 'the sentence is normal'. And precisely because 'it carries normality within it', it has obvious shortcomings when attempting to describe anything that lies outside of the 'norm'. As Brendan Stone (2004: 50) put it, 'Madness is, after all, defined by its difference from reason, and also, to some extent at least, by its variance from the readable forms of narrative.' So to my regret I have somewhat vaporized the seemingly illogical and the affect in the extracts; and the depths and richnesses of how people see and experience the world are limited in their portrayal. Neutered too is the texture of pain and the sensation of the inchoate, as I have inevitably 'pressed' a coherence and form upon the stories – and loss is heavily implicated in this process. As observed by Kathy Charmaz:

> Imposing a narrative frame on research participants' experience may mask rather than illuminate its meanings, particularly those of suffering. From a participant's perspective, the raw experience of suffering may fit neither narrative logic nor the comprehensible content of a story.
>
> (2002: 303)

There were a great many things told to me in the course of the interviews about the very dark sides of living with mental illness and the often tragic, frightening upbringings and life events people had endured. I cannot help but think back to a story of over an hour in length given by a woman who detailed each instance of racist persecution she had faced on her housing estate – reminding us again that people's suffering needs to be perceived intersectionally. Attacked by racists; medicated by doctors; hunted by Home Office immigration enforcement officers; clung to by a terminally ill son; haunted by nightmares – Mercia remarked towards the end of the interview how her creative work not only offered some small relief from her copious skin picking and self-harming, but one day helped her to realize that enough was enough:

> *I thought then, actually I am not going to allow anybody to treat me like that. I don't deserve to be treated like that. I am a creative person, an intelligent person and I am worth every breath that I take.*

In the words of novelist Lionel Shriver (2010: 543) 'Anger generates narrative drive.'

This book is aimed at showing the life-affirming ways in which people come to terms with such histories – sometimes via great detours into anger – and by which they make creative sense of them. It therefore deliberately withdraws from giving much room to the many narrative tracts which elaborate on the pain of people's lives. It is important, however, that in this inevitable process of selection the darker side of people's life trajectories not be undermined. I urge the reader here to bear in mind that behind the sometimes upbeat, often funny, frequently reflective, always generous stories presented here, was a person, not a diagnosis. That person may well have been through – or in many cases is still going through and perhaps will *always* go through – periods of grim despair; painful mental illness; bleak self-doubt; paralysing rage and imploding emptiness.

What I have tried to do is listen carefully within the context of a relationship, however brief – and question how the narrative may be functioning for each speaker, without casting too sceptical a light on narrative 'truth' or the function of a given performance. People told me about their art and their illness, and through whatever levels of promotion, performance, reproduction of discourses, denials or disavowals were being operated, a story of sorts came through; about that person and her journey and about how people narrate their way through dissonant processes of their life. It was precisely *how* these dissonant processes of illness, stigma, symbolic identity theft, abuse, silencing and violence were worked with and narrated through people's art practice that fascinated me – and fascinates me still.

But is it art?

This book is about what people have told me about their art practice; how they got into making art, how they now make art, what their relationship is to that art making, and, sometimes, about the art pieces themselves. There is no value judgement made by me about the 'art' and I do not pass comment on either the aesthetic or commercial value of any of the works. Of course, amongst the pieces shown to me I have my favourites; pieces that moved me or thrilled me or unsettled me or made me wonder at beauty, colour, involvement or movement, or the curious juxtaposition of a found object with a made – but I have deliberately refrained from applause or critique of any of the pieces. Neither do I question what constitutes an art 'practice' – amongst those who spoke with me are people with several exhibitions under their belt and people whose art has never left the confines of their kitchen. What I was more curious about was what each of these levels of practice meant for the makers. As I explore in Chapter 3, I was also interested in what hindered or facilitated the art moving from hospital to public wall or from kitchen to gallery, if that was the aspiration.

Similarly, although there is a brief foray into the literature on creativity in Chapter 2, the words 'creative' and 'creativity' that flowed in and out of conversations I had with art makers are not held up to ideological and discursive scrutiny as they appear in the narratives. Not only is it beyond the scope of this book to enter into the terrain touched on in Chapter 2 in which the discourse of creativity and the tools with which we measure or define it are hotly debated; it is beyond my *intention*. The people who spoke to me about their creative moments, outputs and aspirations had no hesitancy in employing such terms to describe that urge or capacity which gave them vitality and access to worlds and meaning beyond the humdrum. Their ideas of what it meant to be creative chimed with Psychology Professor Arthur Cropley's suggestion that 'the essence of creativity is going against the crowd' (2010: 8). And whilst this arguably simplistic definition defies the deep and complex nature of creativity, it nevertheless provides a window onto how creativity functions in people's lives. Part of this tendency, ability or even need to 'go against the crowd' had, according to many stories, helped people navigate the psychiatric system; confront stigma; cope with family disappointment and even rejection; face the loss of health and material comfort – and turn these life experiences into art. I'd say that was creative.

Neither did participants hold back from describing how mental ill health both damaged their creativity and at times seemed to enhance it. Nor did they shy away from graphically narrating the deadening effects on their creativity of medication, poverty, structural inequality and the psychiatric treadmill. The narratives themselves, I hope, say what needs to be said about creativity within the bounds of this book. It is highly valued; it allows one some means by which to find a way through dark tunnels; it enhances the metacognition needed to see a dark tunnel for what it is; it leads to a product, be it a project, a canvas or a new identity, that, in its making and apprehending, opens vistas.

In the same vein, neither do I enter into descriptions of the art encounter, of how the art that is made impacts, or may impact, on the audience. The nature of the art encounter is again a hugely valuable research direction, regrettably beyond the scope of this book. Nor do I, finally, present descriptions from the narratives of how people felt other art works impacted on *them*, although this would also seem to be a subject worthy of further elaboration and investigation, and necessary to any deeper understanding of the role of the arts in health and wellbeing.

Selected understandings, words and images

When I watch people deeply involved in making art, or when I am at an exhibition watching people looking at the art, there is a *look* on their face. That look speaks of the ineffability of art and its enduring power. How we choose the tools with which to chip away at the ineffable, whether the ineffable delights or distresses us – indeed whether we regard something as ineffable at all – are all questions which for me lie with our 'subterranean researcher' – the one we carry concealed, the one who we only learn a bit about through doing the research.

Oscar Wilde quipped that 'it is what you read when you don't have to that determines what you will be when you can't help it' – and although there is a brand of epistemic plurality in this book, I have particularly mined psychoanalytic theory, because it is to that I return time and again in a motion of homecoming but also a mood of both awe and suspicion, recognition and unease. It is that canon with its sometimes infuriating sagacity that seems to be most equipped to look at the ineffable and the enduring. Psychoanalysis also offers up its words – its language for hurt and trauma; for silences, betrayal and the work of psychic repair. It is, in the words of Michael Eigen (2005: 51), 'a language of wounds'. And I hope that some of the theory and language brought into the following chapters will offer up tantalizing bites of that theory. Bites which urge the reader to explore literature beyond this book through which to enrich their own investigations into the power of making art – this ineffable and enduring thing – and the ways in which it helps us to mend and helps us to grow.

British psychoanalytic theory, much of which falls under the umbrella of the British Object Relations school, offers for my money the most tantalizing clues as to how the human psyche strives unconsciously to repair and to connect; a formulation which speaks well to an understanding of creative activity as therapeutic, life-enhancing, and autobiographic. Kleinian theory and its later elaborations (see Glover, 2009 and Gosso, 2004) offer explorations of art and its relation to the inner world and mental wellbeing of people which are sophisticated, at times opaque, yet also have a kind of common-sense appeal. It stanchly positions the human psyche as social by nature; object-seeking and resilient, not only able to repair damage, but *compelled* to repair damage. It strangely chimes with some aspects of contemporary positive psychology, but offers the theoretical foundations in which positive psychology is still somewhat lacking. So reader, don't stop your searching here.

Throughout this book the terms 'mental illness' and 'mental wellbeing' are used as broad terms to describe conditions that people experience. Some participants have been vocal about preferring the words 'mad' or 'madness' whilst others have objected to there being any particular term attached to what they see as alternative ways of being in, and perceiving, the world. For others still, a specific diagnosis of, say, bipolar disorder, had come as a relief. Some were comfortable with using their diagnosis and diagnostic terms as placeholders – as a means by which to clarify and locate their experiences. So I have used diagnostic terms, but sparingly – attributed usually to people who had used them first in their descriptions of themselves and who referred to the terms as integral components of their identity.

In terms of the images that appear in this book, they were to some degree mundanely determined by our limited space and black and white production. A great many more were generously offered by the artists in this book which could not be shown, and readers are directed to the many varied internet sites where the work of artists with mental health difficulties can be seen, enjoyed and purchased. Artists whose words and work appear in this book were invariably struggling with sometimes severe financial burden, indeed, in many cases, poverty. Such artists will appreciate your support, and potential royalties from sales of this book will be going to the organizations that support them.

> *The security guard knocks on the wire mesh glass window of the door and signals his watch. 'Time is up, Chris', I say. 'See you next week?' Chris nods and compliantly begins to pack Kandinsky away for another week. His features begin to slacken. He'll go back into the TV lounge with its heat, blaring sound and greasy-armed armchairs. 'Till next week, then.' He nods.*

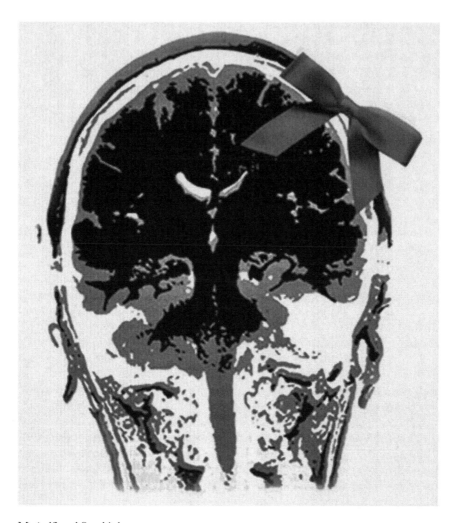

My 'self' and Sarah's bow

2 Mental illness and creativity
Links, myths and arty facts

> . . . the DSM is a work in progress. Within weeks of the appearance of DSM-III in 1980, people were discussing what DSM-IV should look like. After DSM-III came DSM-IIIR (R for 'revised') in 1987, DSM-IV in 1994, DSM-IV TR (TR for 'text revision') in 2000, and now DSM-5. Some suggest that there will never be a 'DSM-6', on the grounds that the whole endeavour is self-destructing.
>
> (Ian Hacking, 2013)

On my shelf I have a musty, 1903 edition of *The Insanity of Genius*. Its inside page is signed in a beautiful but totally illegible hand, and I sometimes wonder at the identity of this long-ago owner. I bought it for less than a quid many years ago, when my interest in the subject was first piqued. On page 317 the venerable J.F. Nisbet, its author, reassures us with the dictum that 'nature is rich in compensations'. If you have the disadvantage of being afflicted with a mental disorder, the idea runs, then nature will endow you with an aptitude or ease in another area of your physical or mental being. Nowadays this might be framed under the rubric of the expanding field of evolutionary psychiatry (see *inter alia* Akiskal and Akiskal, 2005) whereby, it might be argued, genes that cause a predisposition to, let's say, bipolar disorder, are maintained in the gene pool because the creative benefits of the disease weigh against its elimination (Goodwin and Jamison, 2007). In 1997, to give one example, Preti and Miotto proposed that psychopathology traits act as 'hitchhiker engines' able to support the endurance of mental illnesses in the general population, as these very traits are linked to adaptive mechanisms in the species. Such forceful hypotheses have helped sustain explorations into the 'payback' of mental illness. One such payback, our favourite, is that of a possible correlation between insanity and creativity.

Prevalent in popular psychology, the idea of such a link has found its way into our everyday thinking. You may well have shared in exchanges where someone's 'artiness' has been linked, conversationally, to their being 'a bit different'. When I was a teenager, this supposed correlation was a refuge. Instead of seeing myself as the social misfit I was, my moodiness, lack of interactional grace and disdain for the common range of teenage interests of the time could instead be explained away through my avid interest in 'art'. Art – its practice, its discourse, its flamboyance, even its gorgeous smells and paraphernalia – offered an alternative, liminal space to a disgruntled seventies teenager, and throughout history it has been a similar gift to many, who, for whatever reason, have struggled with the mainstream. As narrative extracts in later chapters of this book suggest, however, this gift of art is more openly available to some than to others.

The collapsing of identities – arty/different, or creative/mad – is also a double-edged sword. As with any 'identity' or label, whether we have a role in its choosing or not, it behaves thereafter to confine us, limiting our choices, prescribing our behaviours and delineating how others see us – or indeed do *not* see us. In the words of the Danish philosopher Søren Kierkegaard, 'once you label me, you negate me'. Many of the artists with whom I spoke described such negation, and their battle with labels, categories and the unyieldingness of their walls. Zot Dow, for example, emphasized:

> *I'm an artist, first, who struggles with mental health issues, second. That does not make me a 'mental health artist'.*

I will come back to this act of how participants define the artist that they are in Chapter 3. I will talk further about how the identity and positioning of the mentally ill artist, through discourse, confines practice and maintains barriers between 'high' art and 'outsider' art. But for now, I want to look at how the term 'outsider art' has been arrived at, and to do that I need to meander through the history of the idea that creativity and madness are in some way joined at the hip.

The varied and rich literature exploring a possible link between creativity and madness is usually traced back to the Ancient Greeks. Plato, Aristotle and other Greek thinkers all made reference to such a link in their now much repeated (and sometimes reworked) aphorisms. Roman Stoic philosopher Lucius Annaeus Seneca (c. 1 BCE–CE 65) also linked creative genius to the melancholic temperament. His oft-quoted dictum – 'nullum magnum ingenium sine mixtura dementiae fuit' ('there never has been great talent without some touch of madness') – nestles amongst a clutch of famous references frequently drawn on and cited in support of a perennial link between talent, genius or creativity and madness. Having an idea of the longevity of this link will help frame what follows in this book and will nudge us to question the stereotypes which we all harbour and reproduce about the mentally ill artist.

Madness and creativity: the making of the story

Even a cursory glance at the history of the purported link between madness and creativity quickly reveals two main problems. First, there was, until Michel Foucault in the early 1960s, no consistent critique of the structural forces at play in creating the persona of the mad artist and in enabling incipient creativity to emerge. Even today's studies frequently omit to address the confounding variable of socioeconomic status as pointed out by Waddell in 1998, and there is an implicit message embedded in much of the literature that art somehow transcends class, culture, disability and gender.

The work of art historians Roszika Parker and Griselda Pollock (1981) demonstrated how, for example, women artists have been hindered in their work and written out of history, but there has been little similar attempt at demonstrating how the art practice of mentally ill artists is often thwarted by poverty and the effects of it, both physical and mental. We choose instead to focus on those noble individuals who make art despite their illness, and often despite their poverty. While not wishing to undermine such achievements, focusing on such stories preserves the myth that art and creativity are magical, unbounded forces which will break through the shackles of structural inequality. Such a story tends to backdrop even those studies on the nature of a link between mental illness and creativity deemed 'scientific'. Especially noticeable is the lack of acknowledgement in many contemporary studies that men and women have different rates of diagnosis in some areas of mental ill health (World Health Organization, 2002); that people from low socioeconomic backgrounds are more likely to suffer mental illness (Royal College of Psychiatrists, 2010); or that certain ethnic groups remain over-represented in psychiatric hospitals (Quality Care Commission, 2010). So to talk about a link between creativity and mental illness, we need to ask of the literature, at the very least, whose creativity and whose mental illness are being studied.

Secondly, part and package of the contentious debate about madness and creativity is a lack of clarity and consistency in language and terminology, definition and interpretation. Any attempt at following the thread of claim and counterclaim needs to be mindful that there are only limited instances of convergence of meaning. The very terms 'madness' and 'mental illness' have meant, and continue to mean, very different things to different people. To offer one example, anthropologists Arthur Kleinman and Byron Good, in their 1992 volume on depression, demonstrate how just *one* condition – depression – is so very differently experienced, perceived, spoken of and indeed treated, in different cultures. Their work, amongst others that offer a cross-cultural perspective, serves to remind us of the ethnocentric lens through which we commonly view mental illness.

Mental illness has also meant different things at different points in history, as structures of power have determined the experience of madness at different points in history. Also, the parameters and symptoms of any given condition change as both our discourse and our medical and psychological knowledge evolve – think, for a moment of the transition of the term 'manic depression' to 'bipolar disorder' (Healy, 2008) and the changes attending this transition in our mental imagery, popular understanding and treatment of its symptoms and experiences.

Mental illness categories are constantly in flux, and disorders can only exist in contemporaneous social contexts. The process by which madness came to be redefined as an illness, and hence as a condition that sat almost exclusively within the remit of the medical profession, remains contentious (see Szasz, 1960, 1974). Psychiatry busily redefines terms, creating new illnesses and retiring others; think now of homosexuality, considered an illness until the late twentieth century, only now emerging from the damage of pathologization. Art(istic) and creative(ity), let alone 'genius', are also value-laden terms, without clear definition, and predicated upon temporal and cultural assumptions. The Ancient Greeks, for example, saw genius and beauty as wedded to notions of god(s) and the divine. Plato compounded creativity and madness in his claim that creativity is a 'divine madness . . . a gift from the gods', followed by Aristotle in his 'Problemata xxx' as he wondered pensively about the prevalence of melancholia in those 'eminent in philosophy, poetry or the arts'. Madness seen as an inspiration from the gods, however, still enjoyed a far more positive image than it would in the later centuries to come.

Tacit connections of madness to the divine still hold some sway today – particularly in some cultures. What has become more normalized, however, since the Ancient Greek preoccupation with the subject, is the belief that inspiration and creativity require a dipping into *irrationality* – perhaps in order to access unconscious symbols and thought; an idea to which this book will turn again during its course. This belief in the potential fruitfulness of accessing the subterranean has been the foundation on which contemporary developments of the story of madness and creativity were built.

After the witch-hunts and horrors of the Middle Ages with their formulations of madness based on a frenzied Christian theological mix of the divine, the diabolical, and the depraved, the Age of Reason was to guarantee that great weight was placed on rationality. By the end of the seventeenth century, madness was increasingly seen as an organic physical phenomenon, no longer involving the soul or moral responsibility, and this shift heralded the beginnings of a medicalized discourse which would eventually recast madness as 'mental illness'. The new cult of reason was to ensure the rise of asylums for the insane, and the affirmation that madness, far from being a path to higher states, was in fact an *in*ability to participate meaningfully in the society of the day. Thus the mad required incarceration, and the proliferation of work houses and poor houses – in short the *institution* – was one response to the rise of new social relations. In these relations, families, the fodder of the developing industrialized economy, were now less able to look after relatives in need. With this disciplining of the workforce came intolerance of those falling outside and of those less obedient, compliant, or able. Work houses and poor houses, some of which contained a ward exclusively for 'lunatics', acted as a means by which paupers, prostitutes, orphans, invalids, the old, beggars, the criminal and the mad could be corralled and subdued. Foucault has famously argued that such institutional confinement was based on a condemnation of idleness and an articulation of the imperative of labour, and that it expressed an emerging normative order of modern society and a switch from punishment of the body to punishment of the mind (Foucault, 1995). Thus we arrive at a focus on the 'productive citizen' and the proposed relationship between being busy in the labour force, being included in society and being sane – a focus which was to endure. Similar ideas were to form the backbone of UK inclusion and welfare policy from the end of the twentieth century on.

But confinement, Foucault argued, also effectively robbed madness of features previously empowering, tearing it from its 'imaginary freedom' (1967: 60). In ending the *dialogue* with madness that the Renaissance had maintained, madness was depleted. It was reduced to inhumanity and absence. Relegating the 'mad' to an 'absence' remains one mechanism via which societies continue to 'manage' our anxieties and lack of understanding about mental illness. A further mechanism of 'othering', whereby the mentally ill are objectified and depersonalized, also persists, and has been described by MacCallum (2002), amongst others, as ethically problematic. The mentally ill thus oscillate, throughout history, from being invisible to being othered to being spectacle.

The asylums ushered in new thinking about possible 'treatment', and mechanisms of restraint and control made liberal use of straitjackets, chains, handcuffs and iron collars. Treatment aimed at 'remedying' the insanity included medieval favourites such as bloodletting, purging, the application of leeches, and technological innovations such as gyrating chairs, thought to increase blood to the brain and restore equilibrium. Some forms of treatment were to emerge in direct reaction against the cruelty of accepted practices, and a 'latent humanity emerged among clinicians' (Millon, 2004: 85). Towards the end of the 1700s what became known as the Moral Treatment Movement began to advocate kindness towards the mentally ill, along with purposeful activity. There are echoes of this movement in today's 'therapeutic communities', originally established by, amongst others, Italy's Franco Basaglia (1924–1980). The French physician and philosopher Philippe Pinel (1745–1826) and the English Quaker William Tuke (1732–1822) recommended that treatment should include the use of literature, music, physical exercise and, of course, work. It was suggestions such as these that were to lead in Britain to post-war industrial therapy in psychiatric hospitals, where patients undertook industrial sub-contract work, and to modern-day occupational therapy practice.

The very beginnings of art as therapy were soon to be whispered, in the early nineteenth century. In his treatise *Rhapsodies on the application of the psychic cure method*, published in 1803, the German physician Johann Reil, who was to be accredited with coining the term 'psychiatry', describes an elaborate programme for the treatment of mental illness. This treatment included 'the use of "therapeutic theatre", work, exercises and art therapy' (cited in Ellenberger, 1994: 212). The stage was set for the more widespread, albeit gradual inclusion and therapeutic use of purposeful activity and the arts in the treatment of the mentally ill.

Mad art – an interest emerges

So although the regime for those deemed mentally ill still included routine bloodletting, purging, cold baths, spinning boards and so-called 'tranquilizer' chairs, the nineteenth century heard the creaks and groans of slow change. With the change in activity and treatments that were prescribed for the incarcerated came a growing interest and closer observation of the lives that had previously elicited so little actual interest or concern. Observations of the art making of the 'mad' started to be made.

Philippe Pinel has been credited with being the first to write about the art of the mentally ill, in his 1801 *Medical Treatise on Mental Disorder or Mania*. In this treatise he mentions two patients who drew and painted and also notes his observations of the 'periodic or intermittent' course of manic illnesses. This observation offered an early foray into what was to become a fertile area of research into creativity and mania, and a strand of study in the field very much pursued in psychiatry today. Pinel stands out amongst psychiatrists of the time both for being interested in the *course* of mental illnesses and in his belief in its treatability.

In 1810, John Haslam, from the Bethlem Hospital, became probably the first clinician to reproduce patient work in his *Illustrations of Madness*. In this, the first book-length case study of a single patient in British psychiatric history, Haslam's reproduction of the drawing of his patient James Tilly Mathews was used, however, to support his argument that Tilly was insane, rather than to draw a connection between art and insanity. In 1812 physician Benjamin Rush, who later came to be known as the father of American psychiatry, put forward his suggestions for the treatment of mental illness, and published his inquisitive observations in his *Medical Inquiries and Observations upon the Diseases of the Mind*. In this he noted that 'two instances of a talent for drawing, evolved by madness, have occurred within my knowledge' (Rush, 1812: 152).

Another pioneer of Moral Treatment was the psychiatrist William A.F. Browne, who in 1837 penned the radical manifesto 'What Asylums Were, Are, and Ought to Be' and was an ardent advocate of artistic activity. He initiated a very early collection of patient art at the Crichton Royal Institution at Dumfries, claiming that engaging in art had two main benefits: 'it contributes primarily to impart healthy vigour to the body and secondarily, to expel delusions, and to establish that tranquillity which allows and facilitates the operation of rebuke, remonstrance, threats, encouragement or reasoning' (Browne, 1841, cited in Hogan, 2001: 42). Interest in the artistic activity of the mad was ignited – and was to burn on through the ensuing decades. It was already noted, however, that despite such forward thinking, of all the Crichton patients, for example, only a very small percentage, 3.6 per cent, or forty-six patients, were actually involved in producing art. Of these only ten were women and five were from the 'pauper class' – art was reserved, it seems, for the 'educated' classes amongst the patient group (Park, 2010).

With a belief that idleness has a negative impact on mental states, an ushering in of routines of occupation, activity, and exposure to fresh air and artistic activity amongst the insane was first tolerated and then encouraged. That said, Foucault again critiqued this step change in thinking about and treating madness, arguing that it substituted terror and physical oppression with repression, forcing the mad into regimes of moral obedience predicated upon the standards of a particular social class and religion. This view was contested, however, for its failure to fairly assess psychiatric headway made during this period. Roy Porter (2006), for example, pointed out that Foucauldian zeal tended to obscure the actual progress of humanitarian treatment of the mentally ill. This dichotomy in the thinking of treatment for the mentally ill, with, on the one hand, a belief that treatment represents the end-product of oppressive state mechanisms seeking to subdue and control behaviour deemed inconvenient, expensive or threatening, and on the other, representing a wish to alleviate suffering through utilizing scientific progress, continues to this day. Neither position is clear-cut. But such binary logic does serve to caution us of the potential excesses of each standpoint and the ways in which illness, its perception and treatment are constructed in line with society's discourses and material needs.

In the space allowed by the material progress of the nineteenth century emerged a new breed of asylum doctors, some of whom began to take a specific interest in the artistic creations of their patients. The art of the mentally ill became an established area of interest. The insane artist was once again 'reconfigured' – now as object of academic and clinical interest. Curiosity grew for what the art of the insane might reveal about psychopathology, and later, about art itself, and the role and purpose of creativity as a human propensity. This reconfiguration was to have consequences which continue to reverberate today regarding how art produced by someone with a history of mental illness is received and seen.

The changing economy in the nineteenth century also made possible a free market in the arts in which artists could seek the support of patrons who were no longer confined to the ranks of the church and the aristocracy. It was in the Romantic period, not coincidentally also the period of the industrial revolution, that 'the isolated, private individual appeared on the historic stage' (Oliver and Barnes, 2012: 80). The Romantic movement increasingly looked to madness for unbridled access to exalted states and a way into the hidden realms of the human being. For the Romantic artist, madness held the promise of tantalizing and unexplored realms of the imagination. This other world lay just out of reach, but a small step or twist of the mind into this beyond and through the curtain of 'sanity' could take 'him' into this unexplored enviable terrain.

Romantic artists self-consciously embraced the image of the mad, tortured artist, for the most part conveniently overlooking madness's grim horrors. In selecting and adopting residual cultural and historical knowledge about madness and creativity, and putting this 'knowledge' to the service of a new identity for the Romantic artist, the mad once again came to the service of society, observed through the lens and needs of the time. Becker observes:

> Specific intellectual assumptions regarding creative individuals and the nature of the creative process that the romantics 'inherited' from Greek antiquity, the Italian Renaissance, and the Enlightenment were subsequently transformed into a system of logic that precluded the possibility of total health and sanity on the part of the creative genius. This logic was so compelling, in fact, that self-admissions of mental anguish and actual manifestations of madness on the part of many romantics may be seen as little more than adherence to what had become part of a role expectation deemed appropriate for artists, writers, and other creative individuals.

(2001: 45)

It has also been noted with irony that many of these artists and individuals caught up in the zeitgeist may have been victims of a self-fulfilling prophecy, actually succumbing to a variety of symptoms of mental illness if not full-blown psychosis.

The consumption of opium at the time may have played its part in this, and the occurrence of dual diagnosis (mental illness and substance abuse) to this day can be a confounding factor in research into mental illness and creativity (Mula and Trimble, 2009).

It was the physician Cesare Lombroso, amongst the first to form a collection of the art of the insane, who was to first pioneer actual study into a link between creativity/genius and madness. Lombroso, commonly accredited with being the father of criminology, argued, in his 1891 work *The Man of Genius*, that artistic genius was a form of insanity. He saw insanity as representing a regression to an earlier, more savage stage of human development. There was a link, he claimed, between genius and madness, concluding that both the madman and the genius were types of 'degenerate'. In making this claim, Lombroso drew on the work of French physician Benedict Morel (1809–1873), who, in 1857, proposed a theory of 'hereditary degeneracy'. This biblical idea of degeneration held that people were to be considered 'degenerates' if they were savages or mentally ill because they represented a fall, a *degeneration* from Eden's perfection, as a result of sinful behaviour. An influential concept at the time, the term was attached to all the unwanted, be they children, peasants, women, labourers, or the insane, leading to many of these being condemned and incarcerated. Degeneration theory was to have some staying power as a tool of social control, and, although it was to fall from popularity by the time of the First World War, some of its tenets endured in the world of eugenics and social Darwinists. Lombroso's student, Max Nordau, was to disseminate and expand on Morel and Lombroso's ideas through his own 1892 volume 'Degeneration'. This was to later inform the Nazi wholesale condemnation of 'degenerate art' – just one example of the 'use' to which theories which conflate madness, creativity and a regression to humankind's unbridled passions or instincts have been put.

Lombroso's book is littered with outlandish claims and a zeal for what was to become a further strand of the study into creativity and madness – the search for identifiable characteristics of the art of the insane. In looking for distinctive features in the art of 108 patients whom he considered to show artistic tendencies, Lombroso 'found' recognizable characteristics of the art of the insane, which included 'eccentricity', 'symbolism', 'minuteness of detail', 'obscenity', 'uniformity' and 'absurdity'. He was one of the first, but certainly not the last, to rummage through the imagery of the mentally ill to identify commonalities in the aesthetic qualities of their art. Later, in the twentieth century, Rudolph Arnheim would continue the search for identifiable characteristics of the art of the mentally ill, and the journey to develop a rating scale for a systematic categorization and analysis of characteristics of this art would also get underway (Wadlington and McWhinnie, 1973). Through the twentieth and into the twenty-first century, studies would continue to speculate on what, if any, were identifiable characteristics in the art of the mad (Cohen, 1990; Hacking and Foreman, 2001; Hacking *et al.*, 1996) or characteristics of the mad in the art (Murphy, 2009). Outcomes of these studies are speculative, although at times they have been presented with certitude and fervour.

The nineteenth century would offer up further seminal works ensuing from the rising interest in the art of those deemed mad. In 1907, a French psychiatrist, Marcel Reja, published a pioneering work entitled 'The Art of the Insane' in which he claimed that the art of the insane provides us with a way into understanding creativity more generally. But it took Hans Prinzhorn (1886–1933) and the twentieth century to elevate the debate. Around 1909 he began assembling a small, unique collection of creative works from psychiatric hospitals at the psychiatric department at the University of Heidelberg. Prinzhorn was a psychiatrist and an art historian, a rare combination which was to fuel the enthusiasm from which sprung his 1922 illustrated book, *Artistry of the Mentally Ill*. This book, which focused primarily on schizophrenia as it was then known, took as its organizing line of enquiry 'the border between psychopathology and artistic composition' and sowed the seeds for contemporary investigations. The collection drew on works created by both trained and untrained mental patients, and spoke of what people who suffer from a mental illness create rather than what artists (who may be mentally ill) create.

Prinzhorn opened the way for a fusing of disciplines, using psychoanalytic theories to present the cases of individual artist-patients. He also, for the first time, linked the art of the mentally ill with that of children and folk artists, and this idea was to run, sped on by the French painter Jean Dubuffet (1901–1985). Dubuffet was deeply impressed by the art of schizophrenic patients he encountered on his journey in 1945 to the mental asylum of Waldau near Berne, which had been created far from the artistic mainstream. Dubuffet felt he was observing expressions of an extreme individualism, free from all social and cultural constraints. It was raw – hence his coining of the now well-known term 'Art Brut'. Translated by Roger Cardinal in the early seventies as Outsider Art, the term, its controversies and indeed the market for its artefacts survive; in fact thrive, well into the present day. An umbrella term 'for everything that is ostensibly raw, untutored and irrational in art' (Rexer, 2005: 6), Outsider Art continues both to offer an identity and genre for the work of the mentally ill, but also to delineate and stereotype, as some of the narratives we encounter in this book will affirm.

The association of the raw and the primitive with madness and the relationship with folk, primitive and children's art was an association exploited by both the Surrealists and the Expressionists. The artist Paul Klee, in a diary entry from 1912 where he logged a visit to an exhibition of Kandinsky's 'Blue Rider' group, reflected on the primordial and the art of both children and the mentally ill. While speaking to us of the spontaneity of such art, such conflation of art with raw passion also fortifies stereotypes of madness as belonging to the untamed, wild and unfathomable – stereotypes which have permeated the media as we know it. Studies of the television portrayal of the mentally ill, for example, still reveal that people who have a mental illness are routinely portrayed as having no family connections, no jobs, no moral code, and no chance of being cured (Wahl, 1995). The lines between wild and immoral, tormented but creative and 'mad' are still blurred in popular iconography.

As the Romantics before them had claimed madness, adding cachet and allure to their art, so the later Surrealists were to seize madness, as the apex of free expression and spontaneous passion, for themselves. This is not to deny the mental suffering of some of these artists which has been well documented, or the beauty and power of their work. But what neither the Romantics nor the Surrealists did was to *articulate* the actual misery and despair of the enduring experience of mental illness. Neither did they point out to those pulled along on the fashionable tide of ersatz madness that fellow human beings were being punished, exiled, marginalized and ridiculed for their illnesses – and that *their* overlooked creative work was sometimes the only outlet for this desperate suffering. That said, as pointed out by Rhodes (2000: 85), the mental collapse of Surrealist poet Antonin Artaud in 1937 and the reality of his psychosis somewhat derailed the 'naïve romanticism' of Surrealist attitudes.

The episteme of madness and its mysteries continued its movement from theology, through philosophy and firmly into the emerging science of psychology. In the early twentieth century Sigmund Freud was developing psychobiography, using this means by which to investigate art and its makers. Freud and his former pupil, colleague and then arch rival, Carl Jung, were to diverge dramatically on their thinking about the purpose and value of art, and its relationship to the mind of the maker and beholder. It was a schism which remains in the background of theories today regarding symbolism and creative expression. Jung, on the one hand, saw the therapeutic potential of artistic expression and the possibly universal power and currency of symbols. His thinking was to directly contribute to the development of art therapy as a discipline, with artist and therapist Adrian Hill coining the term 'art therapy' in 1942. In Hill's ground-breaking work using art with injured soldiers returning from the war he found that practising art helped not only to distract them from their illness but to offer them release from distress through the expression of pain associated with what they had witnessed during the war. Hill was to publish the seminal *Art Versus Illness: A Story of Art Therapy*, in 1945.

For Freud, artistic expression was to be held with some suspicion – if not disdain. He regarded it as the sum of sublimated desire, equating the creative process with neurotic defences (Freud, [1908] 1973). But he was to later acknowledge the shortcomings of psychoanalysis in its understanding of art, famously declaring that 'Before the problem of the [artist], analysis, must, alas lay down its arms' (1927: 177). Before laying down arms, however, if he ever actually did, Freud did for art what he did for many other areas of human life – put it firmly on the couch. While Freud's theorizing on art was at times ambivalent and his interpretative methods may now be considered clumsy, his overall message was positive: art is complex; it enhances our lives, and the work that artists do functions as a reparative force in society. His work provided the foundation for post-Freudian psychoanalytic theorizing, which was to offer up some of the most elegant observations regarding the purpose, role and process of art, some of which will be touched upon in Chapters 5 and 6.

Whilst there has been no desire in psychoanalysis to establish a link between art and madness, its theories have been hugely influential in the discipline of Aesthetics. Under its aegis the study of three overlapping areas can be, and has been, carried out. These areas – the nature of the creative process and the experience and inner world of the artist, the interpretation of art and the nature of the aesthetic encounter – have each been enriched by psychoanalytic thought, and, in turn, have deepened our understanding of the *question*, at least, as to whether a link between art and madness exists. So ubiquitous has this influence been that many of psychoanalysis's basic ideas regarding, for example, the role of the unconscious and possible cathartic power in artistic expression have become part and parcel of popular discourse. As I will later suggest, they seem to still hold some keys to understanding the ways in which art is used by those experiencing mental illness. These ideas, however, like all ideas, are double-edged. They have helped maintain an ongoing belief that madness is linked to art via notions such as inhibition and its lack – frequently associated with forms of mentally ill expression and the image of tortured self in need of an outlet. In such thinking we can detect the shadows of beliefs in the primitive and the savage – so we need to be mindful of how embedded such associations are in our thinking.

By the early 1920s psychoanalyst Melanie Klein was using children's drawings as part of her treatment of children as a means by which to explore inner conflict and the depths of their unconscious phantasy. The early work of the predominantly British School pioneered by Klein, Winnicott and Milner helped to develop conceptual tools with which to look beyond the image or the artefact, and into its creating and the meaning of this creating for the artist. It was also to foreground the positive contribution of unconscious mental activity in artistic endeavour. The tools of psychoanalysis and, arguably, mainly those of the British Object Relations School helped pave the way to increasingly sophisticated ways of thinking about art and its role in connection with our inner worlds and sense of self and other. This thinking has provided us with conceptual tools with which to investigate the relationship between pre-verbal experience, the mirroring and attunement role of the primary caregiver and symbol formation, and explore the very roots of creative capacity, points to which I return in Chapter 6.

Nicky Glover in 2009 pointed out that this British Object Relations School takes a largely Humanistic view, one removed from the linguistically-orientated approach employed by poststructuralists such as Althusser, Derrida and Lacan. One of several schisms in psychoanalytic thought, this particular divergence has had an impact, with disagreement over how the subject (individual, artist, mental health patient) is constituted reverberating across the disciplines. It has led to harsh criticisms of individualism and essentialism in much phenomenological work and influenced how we position, present and indeed read the narratives of artists with mental ill health, a point to which I return in Chapter 4. This schism provides an important touchstone in our framing of the debate about a link between mental illness and art as it determines (amongst many other aspects of the debate) how we think about *agency* and the degree to which an individual or a social grouping can use art to contest and challenge.

Psychoanalytic theory on the creative processes is, therefore, not without its vociferous critics, even from within its own ranks. Its analytic processes have been accused variously of killing off creativity by placing art under its incisive scalpel; of pathologizing the artist and of overlooking and nullifying the aesthetic. But it remains a lively, provocative creed, which, while sometimes looking strangely like the maladies it was supposed to cure, at other times holds out truly compassionate and wise observations on the nature of our inner worlds and the products of these – including art.

This book will re-alight on psychoanalytic ideas and their contents in later chapters, but for now let's move our attention to studies which cast themselves within the medico-scientific tradition, sometimes in direct opposition to psychoanalytic ideas so often critiqued for lacking a scientifically rigorous evidence base. Amongst work which could claim more allegiance with such a base, there is a gamut of studies worthy of mention. Let's turn to a very small selection of this work now.

Mental illness and creativity – the later story scientific

By the middle of the twentieth century the drive to establish a scientific base for a link between madness and creativity had picked up momentum. This was partly due to the medicalization of madness which was now complete (madness as mental illness) and due in part to advances in technology, neuroscience and pharmacology which acted as spurs in the field of medico-scientific study. Our fascination with the question of a link between madness and creativity endured, regularly nourished and re-stimulated as the art world in the mid- to late twentieth century and on into the twenty-first exploded with exhibitions of, and debate about, 'Outsider Art'. This upsurge was to witness a proliferation of artists working on the borders of mental illness and artistic expression. Along these borders sat an increase in autobiographic, auto-ethnographic work and later, the newly positioned 'social arts'. This latter gave rise to art created in collaboration with groups deemed marginalized, amongst which the mentally ill were to figure – a development at which I look more in Chapter 3.

Our cultural landscape of dis/ability was shifting again, and old ways of thinking of illness, disability and madness were looking threadbare. Nosed out was the medical model of disability and ushered in were the social and capabilities models which would inform legislation and force us to recalibrate our understanding of the nature of discrimination and disability in society. At the time of writing, new perspectives were again being sharpened, now in response to societal changes where financial instability and severely reduced public expenditure were to impact again on our health and mental wellbeing, and offer a critique of the disheartening new politics which appeared to be replacing confrontation with consensus (Oliver and Barnes, 2012).

But it is under a clinical rubric that most of the research into a link between creativity and mental illness has been carried out in the late twentieth and on into the twenty-first century, re-energizing the story with new seductive characters and plots. Statistical analyses entered stage left, dense with standardized tests, tables, charts, and loud with a cacophony of academic and medical voices. Amidst such a gaggle it is a tough call for the layperson to disentangle what might be valid, resonant, and useful – and what might be stultifying discourse, vulnerable to misuse, reproducing the creative and non-conformist, the misunderstood, or the ill as voiceless laboratory subject – the statistic.

Psychiatry, in particular, with its 'monologue of reason about madness' (Foucault, 2009: xxvii), is demonstrating an enduring fascination for the topic of mental illness and creativity, investing heavily in its quest to provide evidence for or against a link. Many of the studies within this canon do not invite the readership, let alone critique, of the layperson, depending, as they do, on specialized knowledge. They draw heavily on a battery of tools, measurements, specialist terminology and sometimes obfuscating language. But regularly, we, the non-cognoscenti, are treated to the sound bites that the media pull, often recklessly, from these studies. They typically take up a few minutes on a news programme and a few centimetres of space in newspapers, websites, blogs. Here are a few recent tantalizing bites:

- Creativity is akin to insanity, say scientists who have been studying how the mind works.
- Creativity and schizophrenia use similar brain canals.
- You don't have to be mad to be creative . . . but it helps.
- Mental illness link to art and sex.

Headlines such as these and their distilled and often erroneous following paragraphs are then feverishly picked up through blogs and online forums, continuing the Chinese Whispers effect. These headlines and their progeny invariably mask the complexity of most of the studies behind them. They routinely fail too to mention the limitations of the claims; the sometimes skewed samples in which artists of all kinds are lumped together with scientists and even successful business persons as exemplars of the creative human; the assumptions inherent in the use of diagnostic criteria and the blurriness of definitions of creative pursuits – just for starters.

In her pithy critique of studies which claim to offer evidence of the creativity/ madness link, Schlesinger points out that with regard to such headlines it would be helpful:

> if the public understood that although they use the word significant as a synonym for important, an experimental result that is statistically significant may not be important at all; it might not even be particularly meaningful.
>
> (2009: 70)

On the whole, such headlines serve to perpetuate the viability of the link in the popular consciousness, but also to mask the reality of people's lived lives. In many of these realities mental illness is a daily struggle undiminished by scientific proclamations of hereditary, physiological or neurological connections to a creative propensity. It is a struggle invariably exacerbated by structural inequalities and a lack of access to the tools of any creative activity. Such headlines also point to the shifting role and place of science in our everyday lives. Revered and looked to for a solution to every malaise of post-capitalist society in the hope of a label, a diagnosis and a cure – science is also denigrated and rejected for the light it can sometimes shine on some of our shadowy belief systems. Such thinking makes the popular discourse on art and mental illness bumpy terrain – with the adoption of pet theories evident in commentaries, blogs and testimonials, and a flagrant rejection or silencing out of the many sobering conclusions with which science is also credited.

The complexity and scale of current scientific investigations into the possible link between mental illness and creativity is daunting, and only a summary of the field and its main strands is offered here. It will add to our bird's-eye view of our historical passion for this topic, and help to see how current trends within this body of work filter down into popular imagery and discourse, acting to sustain or modify the image of the mad and the artistic within our communities and practices. This summary enters briefly into the worlds of bio-medical science and psychiatry, worlds which have produced a plethora of studies by biologists, neurologists, neuroscientists, geneticists, psychogeneticists and psychologists. It is a high-octane, invitation-only party, one of jousting and edging towards the trophy – evidence at last of a hard and fast scientific link between mental illness and creativity.

Glazer (2009: 755) suggests that 'it is now generally accepted that the link is empirically grounded' but warns of the 'intrinsic disagreements' regarding both the definition of creativity and the classification of different psychoses, and this tocsin cuts to the chase of an underpinning issue. This issue is that of the licence with which the medical establishment in particular has attributed, diagnosed and labelled – and thereafter 'measured' – and the fallibility of language and inter-pretation. As Schlesinger remarks:

> you cannot collect an assortment of studies with different definitions and assessments of creativity and pathology – each using its own research design, with non-random, specialized, and wildly disparate populations – and then point to the resulting pile as being 'cumulative evidence' of anything, no matter how similar the outcomes may seem on the surface.
>
> (2009: 62)

Waddell, too, in her now dated but still cited 1998 review of twenty-nine studies and thirty-four review articles concludes that the enthusiasm for a link between creativity and mental illness has not 'always been balanced with scientific evidence' (Waddell, 1998: 167). Yet neither her selection of studies nor her interpretations have gone uncriticized (Scharfstein, 2009), and, as with virtually anything written in this alluring but contested field of enquiry, there is always a counter claim quick to step up to the plate which, in turn, re-ignites the case for a link.

Such debates are set to continue as research into genetics, neuroscience and the use of Magnetic Resonance Imaging (MRI) technology make further advances in unravelling some of the biological mysteries of schizophrenia (Shenton *et al.*, 2001), for example, and the long-term effects of trauma (McCrory *et al.*, 2012). It is in one way reassuring, therefore, that contemporary studies have become more circumspect in what they set out to do. Negligent and muddled claims of causality and correlativity have for the most part been reduced. An entire genre of studies has emerged, now confining the scope of its investigation to sub-clinical measures of psychopathology, disputing earlier work which has argued that both 'schizo' and 'affective' elements are included in the creative act (Claridge, 1998). These studies fall broadly into two camps, based, at root, on the historical division known as the Kraepelinian dichotomy, after the German psychiatrist, Emile Kraepelin (1856–1926). He first suggested that rather than adhere to a single concept of psychosis whereby all types of psychoses were seen as surface manifestations of a single underlying disease, psychoses should be divided into two – schizophrenia and manic-depressive psychosis, now known as bipolar disorder. Despite arguments for a reappraisal, this division continues to be adhered to within psychiatry, persevering as the foundation upon which scientific claims about which types of mental illness have the hotline to artistic expression are made.

So here the studies diverge – first those exploring schizotypy, a construct that has emerged to denote sub-clinical, psychotic-like characteristics or an underlying vulnerability to psychotic symptoms (Nettle, 2006; Nelson and Rawlings, 2010; Glicksohn *et al.*, 2001), and secondly those exploring hypomania, related to manic depressive (bipolar) disorders (Akiskal and Akiskal, 1988; Ghadirian *et al.*, 2001; Furnham *et al.*, 2008; Vellante *et al.*, 2011). Santosa and colleagues (2007: 31) are not alone in claims that 'After three decades of research, there is persuasive, if not definitive, evidence linking creativity with bipolar disorders in particular.' Santosa and colleagues found that despite the identified weaknesses of their study, their findings suggest there *was* enhanced creativity within their bipolar sample as compared with the control group, a finding supported by a more recent Swedish study. In this, perhaps the largest of the studies in this area, Kyaga and colleagues (2013) assert that *except* for bipolar disorder, individuals from creative professions were *not* more likely to suffer from psychiatric disorders than controls. Also addressed, albeit inconclusively, was the question of the 'inverted-U' model of the relationship between creativity and psychopathology, raised by Richards and colleagues in 1988. In this, increased severity of symptoms appears to enhance creativity to a certain point, after which stage it begins to diminish. This phenomenon may lurk behind some of the skewed results and claims regarding the suggested link between creativity and mental illness and the results found in at least one other study (Rothenberg, 1990), that mental illness more often than not has a negative impact on a person's creativity. Kyaga's study, however, has been criticized on a number of grounds, not least its broad inclusion of professions within the 'creative industries'.

A further line of enquiry in both these strands is pursuing sub-measures within each sub-measure of psychopathology. One example would be the studies looking at the temperament – creativity relationship with patient populations suffering from euthymic bipolar (characterized by minimal symptoms but a vulnerability for mood dysregulation) compared with those with unipolar major depression, who suffer a consistently low mood (Strong *et al.*, 2007). Such data tells us something about how people with different diagnoses create, and when – both at which points in their diagnosis and at which points in their lives. Ghadirian and colleagues (2001), for example, found that in their sample creativity was at its highest level amongst those moderately, as opposed to severely, ill, echoing conclusions of Rothenberg (1990: 164), that 'all types of mental illness engender anxiety that tends to disrupt creative functioning', and Prentky (2001: 102), who warns that 'As mental illness begins to intrude, creativity typically recedes into the background.'

In a now dated but oft-cited study with a large sample, Ludwig (1995) reported the presence of both schizotypy and bipolar disorders in his sample of 1,004 creative men and women, concluding that members of artistic professions are more likely to suffer mental health difficulties and over longer periods of their lives than people from other professions. The hazards of what Schuldberg (2001: 6) termed 'diagnostic lumping' remain, however. Diagnosed individuals may well be included in a given sample which takes a loose definition of a diagnosis, or indeed the individual may be wrongly diagnosed in the first place. In a 2001 review of the theories which have been used to guide explorations into creativity and madness, Prentky concludes that

> Given the current state of knowledge, it seems highly untenable to conclude that creativity has a greater affinity for manic–depressive illness than schizo-phrenia or vice versa. Psychosis is, without doubt, a highly heterogeneous domain of signs and symptoms. Schizophrenia and manic–depressive illness, the two principle [*sic*] forms of psychosis, are heterogeneous and nosologically complex. As such, it is artless, at best, to suggest that either schizophrenia or manic–depressive illness has a corner on the market of creativity.
>
> (2001: 101)

As these two strands of enquiry proceed, both diagnostic criteria and definitions of creativity shift and realign themselves with new understandings – and new needs. Advances in genetic sciences have opened the way for deep investigations into links between family members, and a branch of clinical research investigating a possible link between mental illness and creativity focuses its efforts on transgenerational factors within both. Kinney and colleagues (2001), for example, investigated the creativity in the offspring of schizophrenic parents. Their study claims to offer 'perhaps the strongest evidence to date in support of the hypothesis that traits associated with increased liability for schizophrenia are also associated with increased creativity' (Kinney *et al.*, 2001: 24). Kinney offers the study in support of the theory that enhanced creativity may be a compensatory advantage for genes for schizophrenia, helping to maintain the gene or genes in the population – a view which brings to mind my dusty Nisbet and his dictum about nature being 'rich in compensations'.

In another transgenerational study Simeonova and her colleagues (2005) offer insights into the creative abilities *and* predisposition to Attention Deficit Hyperactivity Disorder (ADHD) of children of bipolar parents, and Kyaga and colleagues (2013), in the large Swedish study mentioned earlier, also claim to have identified a familial association with overall creative professions for schizophrenia, bipolar disorder and other diagnoses. So even bigger and more enticing questions are at stake, regarding what the *purpose* might be for the human race, of both psychopathology and the protean dimensions of creativity. Daniel Nettle (2001, 2006), for example, writes that the hypothesized persistence of genes that may predispose people to mental illness opens up the possibility of cross-checking for such other 'compensations'. It is a persuasive and seductive thought that while 'madness' is disadvantageous, a link with creativity, which *is* advantageous to the species, may begin to explain the persistence of such genetic traces in the human gene pool. The genetic inheritance and transgenerational traces of mental illness and creativity offer an angle of study less concerned with arguing that such a link exists, than with understanding the nature and ramifications of it.

Nettle emphasizes a distinction between psychosis, or actual madness, and psychoticism, which is the personality dimension that may predict predisposition to psychosis. Predisposition to psychosis, if existing on a continuum, would imply that individuals on the higher-risk end of the scale may also have certain creative tendencies. Nettle and his fellow sceptics highlight the point, however, that while a connection may exist between these two traits, it is not necessarily causal. Eysenck (1978, 1996) also reported that although there is no conclusive evidence for a link between creativity and psychosis, there is, nevertheless, a close *relationship* between creativity and 'psychoticism', later defined as a hypothetical dispositional trait – a view which was critiqued by both Claridge (1993) and Csikszentmihalyi (1993).

A further strand of enquiry into the madness/creativity link attempts to determine which cognitive processes, or thinking styles, can enhance creativity and which, if any, of these thinking styles are prevalent in certain types of mental illness. One view holds that it is the personality roots and soft manifestations of schizophrenic *and* bipolar disorders rather than more severe mental illness that are related to heightened creativity. The cognitive peculiarities such as divergent thinking and lowered latent inhibition – the filtering device that screens out lots of information that comes at us every day associated with schizotypic and hypomanic personalities – may be positively related to different kinds of creative pursuits (Burch *et al.*, 2006). Nettle (2001) elaborated this idea in suggesting that schizotypy facilitates the cognitive, divergent thinking part of creativity, while what he refers to as thymotypy provides – in its manic form – the drive and high mood necessary for creative production. It seems that creative individuals, like schizophrenics, may be capable of a widening of selective attention, which renders them more aware of, and receptive to, experience, with a more intensive sampling of environmental stimuli.

People suffering from schizophrenia are often said to be able to make unusual associations, resulting in over-inclusive thinking where many seemingly irrelevant elements are included. Sass (2001), for example, proposed that people on the schizophrenic spectrum may have cognitive vulnerabilities that allow for the mental flexibility that enables a proliferation of innovative ideas and connections. This style of thought is conceived as deriving from a *failure* in the standard filtering of stimuli by dysfunctional gating systems. Yet one can see how this lack of censorship may be beneficial to creative processes, allowing the thinker to include, imagine, elaborate on and connect many strands of thought and information that others would have filtered out, leaving only the utilitarian and the pedestrian. Miller and Tal in 2007, however, argued against this, claiming that their study undermined the 'creativity-benefit' model as an explanation for schizophrenia's evolutionary persistence.

Recent studies have also started to investigate the neurological mechanisms underlying creativity in psychotic individuals. By using near-infrared optical spectroscopy while individuals were engaged in divergent thinking tests, Brandon Folley, a psychologist at Vanderbilt University, reported that creative thinking causes bilateral activation in the prefrontal cortex – the region of the brain associated with higher-order, abstract thinking (Folley and Park, 2005). Schizotypes, however, are said to show an increase in only right prefrontal cortex activation, which is involved in forming unusual verbal associations during divergent thinking. In *Creativity and Madness*, in which Rothenberg takes a measured view of the link between the two, our attention is drawn to the 'Janusian and Homospatial' cognitive processes, as it is by Ehrenzweig in his still insightful 1971 investigation into the 'hidden' order of art. Both these classics discuss these abilities, through which the creative person is able to contemplate and synthesize apparent opposite or contradictory ideas and to bring into fusion two or more discrete entities. Such abilities appear to be alive in both the creative process and in some stages of some forms of mental illness.

The possible connection between creative output, thinking style, and mood, or affect, while not proving or disproving a link between certain illnesses and creativity, at least put the role of *emotion* and its linkages with thinking back on the research agenda, arguing for a more nuanced view of the impact of affect on cognitive activity (Martin *et al.*, 1993). This area of investigation resonates at last with many of the first person narratives gathered in this book, where individuals have described the sometimes painful states of non-productivity with their low mood and black thoughts, followed by upsurges of energy and enchantment where apparently disparate, unconnected and seemingly random thoughts coalesce through artistic process, into an idea or an image. Such descriptions are laden with emotions of both bleakness and joy – reminding us of the interwoven nature of cognition and emotion; and of emotion and creative pursuit.

The proliferation of studies across a range of disciplines and the eruption of interest in smaller and smaller areas of specialization have inevitably led to a fragmentation of the field. Indeed, as cautioned by Hennessey and Amabile:

> investigators in one subfield often seem entirely unaware of advances in another. This means that research is often done at only one level of analysis – say, the individual or the group – and within only one discipline at a time.
>
> (2010: 571)

In sometimes stark contrast to the statistical analyses of personality types, disorders and thinking styles, there is another enduring part of the literature on mental illness and creativity. This consists of biographic studies which explore the lives of creative people in an attempt to isolate characteristics or tendencies which may provide clues about creative lives, and lives into which mental illness has intruded. Some of these studies have been retrospective, and limited by, amongst other things, decreased reliability due to making diagnoses based on biographical information and *post hoc* diagnoses. This tradition, which arguably began with such retrospective studies as Freud's study of Leonardo and Michelangelo (1910, 1914a), continues to be popular, with contemporary studies throwing light on artists and their (sometimes imaginatively claimed) pathologies. There has been considerable criticism, however, of such *post hoc* diagnoses and ensuing analysis, with Schlesinger (2009) amongst others questioning the validity of psychological autopsies as research tools. Kalian and colleagues (2002: 675), too, cautioned that 'exploiting literary heritage as a tool for postmortem psychiatric diagnosis is rather complicated. Such a study poses both phenomenological argumentation and ethical debate, especially when no reliable psychiatric documentation exists.'

But the fascination for such retrospective study of artists continues (Murphy, 2009), as does the exploration into those still living and *their* predecessors. In his 1970 study of great painters, Karlsson found the ratio of psychosis in great painters to be 35 per cent above that for the general population; Schildkraut and colleagues (1996) reported that affective disorders were ten times more prevalent and the rate of suicidal behaviour three times greater in a group of New York abstract impressionist painters, compared to the general population. Akiskal and Akiskal (1988) in a study of living painters found that 50 per cent had experienced major depressive episodes, while two-thirds had recurrent cyclothymic or hypomanic tendencies. A 1994 study on visual artists and writers by psychiatrist Felix Post showed that 37 per cent of the artists suffered from severe psychopathology and 42 per cent from depression. Ludwig's earlier mentioned 1995 work claimed that certain emotional disorders in female writers suggested a direct relationship between creativity and psychopathology, but cautioned that, again, the relationship was by no means a simple one.

Most often cited and hotly debated (Sass, 2001; Rothenberg, 1990; Schlesinger, 2002) are two studies by Andreasen (1987) and Jamison (1989). Both of these researchers undertook to study a sample of creative individuals with the aim of establishing whether there was any correlation between their creativity and mental illness. Both studies, most notably the latter, remain favourites in the popular imagination, spurred on by a prolific dissemination through online forums such as blogs, and their inclusion on university reading lists worldwide. Such fervent reproduction by, it has been suggested, people who have never actually read the primary source material they are citing (Schlesinger, 2002), adds to what Sass (2001: 77) has described as 'collateral damage' to the 'image and the self-understanding of schizophrenia-spectrum patients' incurred through the 'vigorous pursuit of the affective–creativity connection'. Both studies have come in for criticism of flawed methodology, weak analyses and over-dramatized claims. Rothenberg (1990: 150) points out that in these and other similar studies, 'the need to believe in a connection between creativity and madness appears to be so strong that affirmations are welcomed and treated rather uncritically'. Andrew McCulloch of the Mental Health Foundation reminds us, in his 2012 cautionary critique of such studies, that it is unwise:

> to forget the intense distress these kinds of illnesses can cause, or see 'mental illness' as simply the flipside of a creative mind, the price you pay for being an artist. Anything that trivialises mental illness like this has the potential to be unhelpful and even dangerous.
>
> (McCulloch, 2012)

Both madness and creativity are slippery, contested terms and constructs. The political nature of both terms is revisited in this book, and such visitations release me from an otherwise overwhelming impulse to place 'madness', 'mental illness' and 'creativity' always within the inverted embrace of the 'scare marks'. What many of the studies into a link between mental illness and creativity do, as is evident after even this cursory look at the literature, is remind us of how difficult it is to define the illnesses which come under a category of mental illness or disorder. The 'wholesale comings and goings of disease classifications' (Porter, 2002: 216) of the Diagnostic and Statistical Manual of Mental Disorders (DSM IV) and its critics are, in themselves, testament to the rapidity of changes and uncertainty of knowledge of the area. As this book was being prepared, the DSM had just become DSM 5 and was subject to its most vociferous critiques to date; Ian Hacking's caution at the beginning of this chapter being amongst the more restrained.

But as with 'mental illness', so too is the nature and construction of *creativity* debated. Barron and Harrington begin their 1981 paper with a snapshot of the emergent fields within creativity research, which portrays a burgeoning fascination which has not lessened in pace or scope since:

> Divergent thinking; creativity in women; hemispheric specialization opposing right brain to left as the source of intuition, metaphor, and imagery; the contribution of altered states of consciousness to creative thinking; an organismic interpretation of the relationship of creativity to personality and intelligence; new methods of analysis of biographical material and a new emphasis on psychohistory; the relationship of thought disorder to originality; the inheritance of intellectual and personal traits important to creativity; the enhancement of creativity by training; these have been the main themes emerging in research on creativity since the last major reviews of the field.
>
> (1981: 439)

Koh (2006) gives an analysis of how both terms, mental illness and creativity, have changed and been changed by the advent of postmodernism, and how this colours the ways in which we think of, categorize and study each. Sass (2001) has suggested that a 'romantic' conceptualization of creativity fits with affective temperaments, while a postmodernist view of creativity defined in terms of hyper self-consciousness fits better with schizophrenic tendencies. He also warns that:

Creativity is not, after all, the most unproblematic or transparent of theoretical constructs. Despite the surprising confidence of some psychologists and psychiatrists who write on the topic, it seems unlikely that the term creative refers to a single, underlying essence or that its application can be separated from culturally determined and socially generated forms of interpretation and evaluation.

(Sass, 2001: 55)

Questions about the nature of creativity, or what Nettle (2001), after Shakespeare, referred to as 'strong imagination', have far from abated. Technological advances and more refined excavation into the philosophy of aesthetics have, unsurprisingly, raised the bar since Rothenberg's (1990: 4) statement that 'there is little consistency or definite agreement about the meaning of the idea or of the specific term "creativity"'. Eysenck (1996) defined creativity as the ability to produce ideas, insights, inventions or new or original art products, accepted by experts as scientifically, aesthetically, socially, or technically valuable – and indeed some creativity studies have investigated creativity as expressed through scientific, technological or even business and commercial endeavour – sometimes, problematically within the same sample.

Creativity, for much of 'human history the prerogative of supreme beings' (Csikszentmihalyi, 1997: 5), like mental illness, poses enduring questions. Is its source located in the unconscious, as claimed by Freud in 1917, or is it 'primary process thinking' driven by basic human instinct and free from constraint, as he suggested in 1958? Or, is it from cognitive processes that novel ideas emerge and are realized? Biological bases are still claimed while psychotherapists such as Anthony Storr (1993) have put forward views that creativity is a product of the infinite adaptability of human nature faced with the need to respond to changing social and physical environments – a proposed link with the pull again of evolutionary psychology. Glazer (2009: 755) in her detailed overview of creativity types and paradigms points out that 'paralleling dimensional conceptualizations of psychosis, the creativity construct could extend along a continuum; or it could exist in different distinct and independent forms'.

In a 2006 study Banaji and colleagues looked at the *rhetorics* of creativity. Although the review focused on work of direct relevance to education, where understandably concepts of creativity are hotly debated, the report serves as a useful reminder that part of the problematic package of what creativity is or might be – let alone who 'has' it or 'is' it – remains the fact that creativity is defined by discourses. Such discourses make judgements regarding aesthetic and cultural desiderata. They function as rhetorical stances, which are organized to persuade and to bring about consensus (Habermas, 1984). Nowhere is this more apparent than in the rhetoric of creativity as economic imperative. Here, the concept of creativity has been politically reconceptualized as a means of responding to broader socio-political and economic agendas and summoned to the service of a neo-liberal economic programme. As Neelands and Boyun Choe (2010: 291) point out: 'Creativity is not a natural phenomenon like a sunset or osmosis. It is a culturally specific construction which is defined so as to serve the interests of particular positions in the field of cultural production.'

We are also reminded, however, that a view of creativity as being essential to social and economic wellbeing goes back to the Chinese Emperor Han Wu-Di who reigned from 141 to 87 BC (Cropley, 2010). And so, like so much in this enduring debate, this harnessing of creativity to the economic machine is not a new idea but one recycled and reconstructed to come to our service in a different moment of social development. What is worthy of note, however, is the now vast range of mechanisms and structures issuing from policy that act on a very practical level to define who gets to be creative, whose creativity is recognized, and to what use it is put. Neelands and Boyun Choe (2010: 292) remark that, 'Put simply, children of certain socio-economic groups are more likely to be recognised as being "creative" than others.'

There are therefore pressing questions about the role culture has played, and does play, in defining both madness and creativity, with suggestions that 'the link between creativity and madness is nothing more than a creativity myth, springing from [the] Romantic era conceptions' (Sawyer, 2006: 87). As Erving Goffman (1963: 138) put it, 'the normal and stigmatized are not persons but rather perspectives', and no less is true of creativity – how we define it, employ it, attribute it, constrain or enable it are driven by one's perspective. In talking about a link between madness or mental illness and creativity we are only ever dealing in perspectives; but before we dissolve entirely into relativism here, let's be mindful that perspectives not only spring from, but support and reproduce particular social orders.

One outcome of the maintenance in the popular imagination of creativity myths has been a continued skewed image of mental illness. Our internal imagery of mental distress is still often allied with notions of the reclusive, impassioned artist – allowing us to circumvent the pain, tragedy and horror of mental illness. Ironically, the creative activity and the sometimes startling products of mentally ill artists often allow us to avoid looking at the *distress*. As Roy Porter (2002: 182) soberly puts it: 'When Van Gogh painted himself, who can say whether he was painting madness? All that is clear is that he was painting misery.' Van Gogh was similarly evoked by Simonton (2010: 229) who concluded that 'However original and exemplary Van Gogh's paintings may be, I would not wish his tormented soul on my worst enemy.'

The regular and automatic link we still make between creativity and madness has a further irony in that its presence in our collective consciousness may actually deter mentally ill people from participating in artistic activity which could potentially contribute to achieving psychological wellbeing because they do not identify with the stereotypical idea of 'mad creative'. The flip side of the coin, however, is that for others who suffer from mental illness, the possibility of claiming an identity as 'artist' may indeed offer the possibility of a more congruent and empowered identity (Gwinner *et al.*, 2010). Both of these positions were echoed in the narratives gathered for this book.

So the idea, the belief, or the myth, depending on one's standpoint, that creativity and madness are inherently linked continues to have a romantic appeal, and for Waddell (1998) there may be yet another reason for the enduring attraction of the link, suggesting that 'both mental illness and creativity have become metaphors for nonrational or spiritual needs that are sublimated in our rational, scientific age'. Whatever the reason, the *schadenfreude*, the comfort, and the alibi of the myth are all too seductive. For now, some argue the jury is out, with Sawyer (2006: 87) maintaining that 'Despite almost a century of work attempting to connect creativity and mental illness, evidence in support of a connection has been remarkably difficult to find.' I will end this brief and scattered journey through the making of the myth with a caution from Waddell:

> We may do more harm than good to the cause of creativity if we inadvertently convey the idea that creativity and mental illness are both forms of deviance. We may do more harm than good to the cause of alleviating mental illness if we romanticize mental illness and trivialize its impact by associating it with creativity. We may do more harm than good if we fail to note that mental illness impedes creativity or if promoting an association between creativity and mental illness takes precedence over either encouraging creativity or reducing mental illness.
>
> (Waddell, 1998: 170)

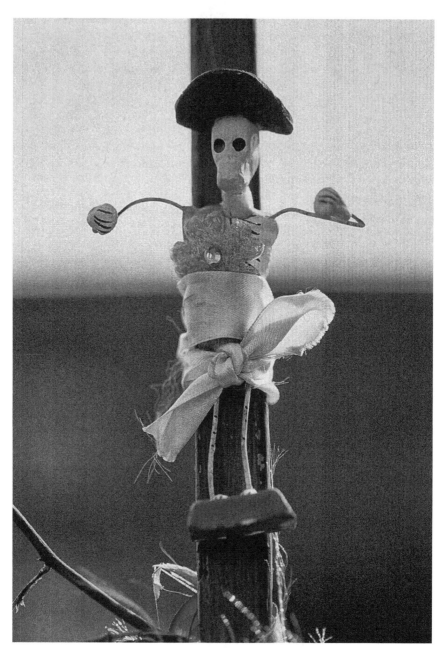

Untitled

3 Transitions

Participation and collaboration

The word 'art' includes a value judgement within its fixed emotional connotations. It sets up a distinction between one class of created objects and
another very similar one which is dismissed as 'nonart.'

(Hans Prinzhorn, 1922)

Twenty-first century. The asylums have been done away with. The infamous
'mental institution' I used to pass as a kid on my way to school has, like many
others, been converted into high-end executive apartments. It boasts its own gym,
tennis courts, landscaped gardens and cleansed institutional memory. I wonder if
the new inmates who swish around its interior give much of a thought for the
wretchedness that must be etched into the very foundations of the imposing
nineteenth-century building.

Through the grassroots movements and activism of the 1960s and 1970s Mental
Health has gradually become stamped with different terms and possibilities. There
has been radicalization and empowerment of the mentally ill through the
Survivor's Movement, the Recovery Movement and Mad Pride; a rash of acts and
policies[1] and a dispersal of those with mental ill health from institutionalized care
into the community, although many argue this latter has had more to do with the
increasing difficulty of justifying the cost of segregation than with humanitarianism
(Scull, 1984). Brief hospitalizations, outpatient care, new anti-psychotic drugs and
a better understanding of illness management strategies have transformed the
ecology of mental illness. Discourses framed by the Social Model, and its progeny
the Affirmative and the Capabilities Approach to understanding illness, have
nibbled away at the dominance of the medical model of disability and illness and
shown us the complexities involved in living with stigma, illness, dis/ability. But all
is far from rosy for those who suffer from mental ill health. A 2010 report by Peter
Beresford and colleagues for the Joseph Rowntree Foundation found that in their
sample of fifty-one mental health service users, most 'believe that a medical model
based on deficit and pathology still dominates public and professional understanding of mental health issues, shaping attitudes and policy'.

Care in the Community, the British policy of deinstitutionalization, has dispersed
the mentally ill into a range of settings and loose nets often largely held together,
some argue, by hope. Homelessness, experienced by so many mentally ill people,

is 'fuelled by a mental health system that fails to provide even rudimentary care for those formerly housed in institutions' (Hinshaw, 2011: xii). The website of the Department of Health for England announces that mental illness is the largest single cause of disability in our society, yet in the UK the Coalition government's main response to the nation's economic problems has largely been to target the support systems of the most vulnerable, the mentally ill included.

There remains, however, a desire within mental health services, amongst service users and policy makers (although reasons behind this desire are by no means always shared), to reframe mental illness and re-envision what rights, care and discourse are appropriate in the post-institutional era (Davidson *et al.*, 2010); a desire to close the doors on the asylum *mentality* once and for all. Franco Basaglia (1924–1980), the Italian mental health reformer, once wondered how, now that we have freed persons from the asylum, persons might free asylums from themselves. And therein lies a continuing task. The implicit asylum mentality of today is steeped in notions of segregation and exclusion, and in a boisterous assumption that integral to normality and sanity is participation. Active participation in a community, in wider society and particularly in the labour force is the current disciplining discourse, a benchmark by which your sanity is evaluated by the extent of your visible participation as a productive citizen. There is some irony in this given the deification of individualism still prevalent in developed Western society, not to mention a difficulty, given the shrinking labour markets and decreased access to community services.

In order to close down the asylum mentality, communities have to be opened up. The twenty-first century has given us high-level campaigns and high-profile celebrity stories which have penetrated the media with urgent messages to end stigma and to see through the stereotypes to the person. We are reminded that one in four of us are likely to suffer with mental ill health at some point – so don't go pointing at a 'them' who may well be an 'us'. Whether this alarming ratio is because of the mushrooming items of the American Psychiatric Association's Diagnostic and Statistical Manual of Mental Disorders (the DSM 5 released in 2013 included a further fifteen new diagnoses); or because twenty-first-century living is more likely to drive us crazy; or because, increasingly reluctant to accept the sadnesses of life we have become more eager to put human dis-ease down to illness; or perhaps because we count some things for the first time, and old things differently – are all debates that continue to rage in the daily exposure of mental illness. Yet despite this exposure and the open debates, the narratives gathered for this book by and large told of experiences of being silenced; of self-censoring to avoid stigma and discrimination; and of having to fight hard to become a presence rather than an absence or a menace. In 2013, the supermarket giant Asda advertised on its website a 'mental patient fancy dress costume' on sale for Halloween. It came complete with fake blood, a mask and a meat cleaver. It was hurriedly withdrawn after an outcry, with Asda promising to make a 'sizeable donation' to a mental health charity, but its brief appearance reignited debates about just how much in the public and corporate imagination had actually been changed about mental health and the prevailing stigma surrounding it. As commented by former political aide and depression sufferer Alastair Campbell, 'Something like this comes along and it just reminds you we are basically still in the Dark Ages' (BBC News, 2013).

The stigma, debates and uncertainties about mental illness, what it is, what each 'condition' is, and, as Ayden put it, 'how I am to configure myself vis-à-vis it' – breathed in people's stories. Oftentimes what people felt seemed to conflict with what they had been told about themselves, and this dissonance set in train an undermining of their own personal experience. When speaking of his illness, Paul, for example, was adamant that his long-term illness was rooted more deeply than in a suggested imbalance of serotonin levels:

> *It's a real depression. It's not a chemical thing. I've taken anti-depressants and they've done nothing for me because they don't address the root of the problem.*

And Ayden veered from confusion to frustration about what he was 'supposed' to have or be – but insisted that the way he felt was at the core of any understanding:

> *I've been diagnosed as depressed, anxious, then bipolar . . . I think earlier they said I had dissociative disorder . . . that I am this, that . . . (sigh) . . . I'm just me, to me . . . (pause) and stuff happened . . . and I know what I **feel** about it . . . I look there.*

Mickie's experience of receiving different and changing diagnoses was shared by many:

> *It wasn't really until I was 21 I had a proper breakdown in the sense that I went to hospital. It really was a breakdown in the sense I just couldn't talk anymore, I couldn't communicate to anybody and so that's my first real experience of what is commonly known as mental illness. And then there was a whole kind of sequence really until I was 32 in 2002. That was the last time I was in hospital anyway, at which time I was diagnosed with bipolar affective disorder, which I suppose it's still a bit shaky. Originally, the first time I was in hospital the doctors thought I was schizophrenic, although they weren't really sure. They wanted me to stay but I was there voluntarily. To be honest, I was frightened in being diagnosed in any way and also very fearful of the whole thing. I just wanted to be normal I suppose.*

It was notable in the narratives that some participants had made several renewed efforts to come to terms with each given label and its implications, researching what each was, its prognosis, medication, possible aetiology, and becoming versed in its descriptors and terminology. Caught up in the 'colonizing discourse' (Dillon and May, 2003) of psychiatry, therapy and self-help, the emerging and persuasive language of neuroscience, and the dispassionate language of the pharmaceutical industry, narratives often revealed the ongoing task of attempting to make sense of an illness and to take possession of a language with which to describe oneself and *be*. Froggett and colleagues (2011: 30) refer to this as language which has lost resonance with lived experience, and indeed in many interviews this experienced dislocation between language and felt experience was explained away by the remark, 'that's why I do art'.

Part of the making of sense was locating oneself within such discourses, or in opposition to them – by developing a counter-narrative; and this chapter and the next look at some of the ways in which this was done. For me, listening to the candid stories that people shared – stories which were often littered with the debris of wrecked childhoods of trauma, abuse, emotional neglect and the later unending battles of the daily tasks of living – left me with an alternative question. How is it that people can be so *sane* having lived such things? For many, that sanity, that continuing narrative of life, was at least partly, and for others wholly, due to art:

> . . . *in a lot of ways, my involvement in the arts is one of the primary things that helps me cope with my depression and my circumstances. It's probably the raison d'être of my life, the primary thing in my life.*
>
> (Paul)

> *Art is the thing that gets me through all the barriers that I get to in my life.*
>
> (Crystal)

It is important, therefore, that the ways in which people with such difficult life trajectories become involved in art be defined, recognized and celebrated, and that mechanisms to expand accessibility to these are embedded in health policy. In these times of shrinking welfare, such ways into art need to be guarded, protected and fought for.

I want to examine in this chapter how people from various walks of life at different life stages and ages and from a variety of cultural backgrounds got to practise their art. How was it that they reached out from within the turmoil of breakdowns, hospitalizations, medication-induced haziness, bleak corridors of depression, prison and homelessness – to paper, to camera, to canvas and to the found objects, the bits of tin and cardboard and debris with which some, in the absence of other materials, worked? What aided or hindered them?

Darrell, recently diagnosed with Borderline Personality Disorder, describes how he started to draw, from within a past of alcoholism, homelessness, petty crime and violence that he has now come to do battle with, in his paintings:

> *It's kept me going. I've been in prison a few times, as I say, nothing major, stupid things – shoplifting, police assault – mostly when I'm under the influence of alcohol, but as I said, I've always ended up in the hospital wing of the prison, because inevitably I've been a bit psychotic . . . or whatever, and the one thing that has always managed to keep me sane, to a degree at least, is that they eventually find out that I've got a bit of drawing talent or whatever and give me some paper and a pencil and I start drawing and that inevitably helps me to recover and I get off the hospital wing and put into a normal wing. So my art has been instrumental in helping me to stay sane.*

Many of the artists who spoke to me mentioned art therapy, community arts, participatory arts or social practice – terms which flowed in and out and through the narratives as individuals described their involvement and sometimes disavowal of such practices. Each was commonly spoken of with some certainty – the narrator had constructed a meaning for each of these and their setting, boundaries and expectations. What is noticeable is how these *ideas* of modes of practice had become lodged in the imaginations of artists, project workers and those involved in 'the community' – and it is worth saying something about how they were perceived and the function each was felt to perform.

Transition: the role of art therapy

For some, involvement in community arts, or art in adult and community learning or higher education, 'happened' through the experience of having art therapy. Strikingly, many people spoke of the ad hoc way in which such therapy was available – many were not offered art therapy as part of their treatment, and expressed regret. Some were offered a short series of sessions, or even a one-off. The quality of the encounter and techniques, materials and settings varied enormously, too, with some people speaking of a sustained and rich relationship with the art therapy, and others being 'given some paper and a few pencils while someone walked around looking in now and again . . .'.

In almost any form, for most who had encountered it, art therapy had provided a welcome relief from the drudgery of hospitalization. For others, it had offered an appealing alternative to talking therapy, which, as I will revisit in Chapter 4, was spoken of as having limitations. Art therapy, it seemed, had provided another significant comma, punctuating and offering coherence in a story away from deep illness.

But, as a practice which traditionally foregrounds the therapy over the art, art therapy was also sometimes regarded by its recipients as 'getting in the way' of the art and the potential development of transferable artistic skills. This view was mostly held by people who had a longer history of making art and, to some extent, felt impatient with what was seen as the 'imposition' of 'psychologizing' on what was a protected area of their life and expression. By far the majority of people with whom I spoke had memories stretching back into childhood of making some sort of art, and they were often adept at making links between what they had produced as children, and their mental health. Here is Chloe Shalini:

> *From very early, I was fortunate enough to be given crayons, colouring books and scrap paper to scribble on from age two or three. I remember being very interested in drawing 'princesses' about age four/five, in my mind not so much royal, as I had no understanding of that, more 'nice girls'. . . . I distinctly remember having image problems from the age of three. I already felt insecure around girls I perceived as prettier, 'nicer' – more 'adequate'. My inspiration for 'princesses' came mainly from books, I was blessed with a lot of those . . . and probably also from Disney! It made me feel better about myself to draw these 'ladies', as I called them. I felt they were friendly, a bit like having imaginary friends. I was also drawing how I wanted to be. I liked to believe I could change and maybe become 'good'. Because, like a lot of abused kids, I thought I must be very bad, and fat and ugly.*

For some of these art makers, it might be that they have less motivation or desire to work with the 'inter' psychic, transferential phenomena of some art therapeutic approaches, and more of an interest in the '*intra*' psychic. A few spoke of having moved from a 'venting' to 'distraction' role for art making (Drake and Winner, 2012), feeling that they had purged what needed to be purged, and that now art functioned as a diversion away from a past, from their illness, from painful memories and thoughts. They felt that the therapeutic process by default committed them to working with the past, one from which they were making a deliberate attempt to move away:

> *I'm done with going over and over the story. I'm done with dark paintings. I want to look at something . . . anything . . . an animal, a flower, something not me, and say 'that's my subject' . . . there's something about that very decision that is important to my being well . . . looking ahead . . . beyond . . .*

> (Leonne)

This dichotomy, between a commitment to exploring the past or making a deliberate move to a focus on the future and employing the cognitive processes necessary to making this shift, echoed throughout the narratives and was sometimes expressed within the same interview. I will be returning to this in later chapters, as it reflects two perspectives within therapy, based on two models of psychological functioning and what processes are involved in recovery and wellbeing, warranting further discussion. For many recipients of art therapy, however, its process of bringing to their attention the meanings which may sit behind the symbols and forms they were producing was a welcome 'light bulb' moment:

> *What I didn't realize is that you then all sit around and discuss the piece of work and I had nothing to say about my work because I didn't think I was emotionally connected to what I had drawn. And then the art therapist started to suggest – not suggest, ask me – if it represented how I felt about my place in the world, being alone on a desert island . . . and I just completely broke down. (Pause). It connected so utterly.*

> (Crystal)

The value of art therapy in the care of people with mental health difficulties is not disputed here, nor is the body of mainly psychoanalytic theory that underpins its practice to be undermined for the insights it offers into people's illness, wellness and the journeys to and from,[2] and this is further explored in Chapter 4. But the identity of service user or survivor is one more autonomous, critical and empowered than ever before. There is less tolerance now than in the past for the inherent asymmetry of power in relationships of therapist and therapized, and more suspicion of the limitations imposed on the 'client' through the discourse of therapy. Joy Schaverien, for example, wrote in 1993 that patients' artworks provide a record of the patient's experience to *add* to that of the art therapist's record. Yet this reveals one of the fundamental problems of art therapy in that the client's perspective remains secondary to that of the therapist. Therapeutic practices, as critiqued by Guilfoyle (2005: 101), may be felt, in fact, to be incapable of 'stimulating effective resistances against culturally dominant discourses and practices'. And it may be for these reasons, amongst others, that hybrid practices such as participatory projects with artists, non-therapy arts projects and Arts in Health[3] projects were spoken of in very different tones, with more spontaneous detail, enthusiasm and greater sense of ownership:

> *In the 80s I got involved with the service user movement. I also at the same time tried to do a course on art therapy which I did for two years but found it very difficult because they used the medical model and the psychotherapeutic model and I couldn't really bring in to it any experiences of psychiatry which formed a big chunk of my life at that time. And so I finished the course, I passed it, but I never practised as an art therapist – I think I had a big conflict between art therapy, because art therapists want people to interpret their work, they want them to be, in a kind of be in a clinical setting . . . to see that it's having an impact on their life, it's somehow changing it and I think it's more for the therapist than the practitioner.*
>
> (Mabel)

The transition from a service user identity often included making a break, consciously or not, from art therapy, which was too easily associated with an unequal clinician–patient relationship and one's *past* identity. It was also seen to be less imbued with possibilities for an emerging artist. Making art was always spoken of as therapeutic, a point I return to in Chapter 4, but one's practice, it seems, had to be wrestled away from the art therapy domain and nurtured in a new setting. That setting needed to offer equality of relations, to be felt to empower, and to position the art as aesthetic, not therapeutic tool. Mabel continued:

> *Instead in my role . . . I suppose as a service user and being involved in the Bridgewave mental health forum, we tried to set up art projects in the Bridgewave area for and with people with mental health problems. In the, well I'm talking about the 90s now, we set up with the social services in a mental health resource centre, the Arts Hub which has really been a huge part of my life, my art development and a contribution to actually changing the services and making them more accountable and more reflective of the needs of people with mental health problems and their own art development . . . we didn't want it to be about art therapy, we wanted it to be therapeutic, enabling, empowering but actually giving people the space to do what they want without having to explain it really.*

The importance of a suitable space and place, one that was felt to be 'safe', was not to be underestimated, a point also found by, amongst others, Stickley (2010). This need for a 'place' to practise, to discuss, make collaborations, display and store one's work was woven into the many stories of the role, in the lives of mentally ill artists, of community arts.

Transition: the role of community arts

By far the most commonly referred to term in the narratives when people spoke of how they accelerated their own practice was 'community arts'. This amorphous category, which can be traced back to the 1960s, is still motivated by an ideology loosely revolving around attention to the marginalized and disadvantaged and collaborative ways of working and empowering peers.

Community arts emerge in the narratives through descriptions of an assortment of practices, venues and objectives; some spoke of belonging to a local group which had sprung up through joint interests amongst people loosely known to each other. Some community art was rooted in a project, or series of projects based in a small gallery, perhaps involving the participation of several people committed to producing one outcome. There were a number of short-term projects generated through colleges and adult services, or joined by the thread of a local hospital or charity, some under the rubric of Arts in Health which included an arts practitioner working in a hospital or mental health setting. These projects varied in their longevity, facilities, funding, and in their levels of connection to other networks and institutions. Some were highly sophisticated operations linked to a university and sponsors, employing paid members of staff. For some, it seemed that their very hybridity was the strength, offering release from confinement in any one 'sector'. As observed by Mike White (2010: 20): 'the secret is to not look at arts as something delivered by an artist or by an arts organisation. It happens best when it comes out of a dialogue between different sectors.'

Whatever the project, or place, 'community arts' was frequently spoken of as having acted as a catalyst or a lifeline of transition. This transition ran from one having an identity of service user or mental health sufferer, to *something else*, a something else which was deemed vital in terms of hope and recovery. The co-founder of one established project, herself an artist and mental health service user, described how pivotal this could be:

> . . . *people who've come to Artstown have moved out of residential care and moved into their own homes and part of that is the . . . coming here, is the socializing, is the being able to express themselves in a different way. But also it gives people a lot of confidence. One of the things that was really amazing the other week we had an opening of an exhibition and for the first time ever somebody was able to bring their wife and their children and suddenly their family could see them as somebody else not as someone who unfortunately has a mental health condition but actually somebody who's capable of doing things and doing things well and they can feel more engaged with . . . and that's quite often some of the feedback we get back from people, that they can start having different conversations with people, they can go out with their friends, they can go out and socialize better. It's very simple running art workshops in a way, enabling people to have that then confidence and kind of ability to talk about something different. The other thing Artstown gives is that most people who come here and make art couldn't afford even some of the most basic things that we give them whether it's canvas, access to paints or even access to books, or exhibitions, you know they wouldn't have it otherwise.*

> (Ruth)

Marty, an accomplished artist in his early forties, both works in, and practises with, community arts groups. He looked back on how community arts gave him a chance to change career and re-define himself:

> . . . *I had my last quite bad depression and decided to change careers and work in mental health, starting as a volunteer with local community art groups* . . .

Still suffering recurring bouts of debilitating depression and still producing a large number of highly detailed, carefully executed paintings and drawings, Marty now works full-time as a mental health services project worker, involved with Arts in Health work. He was not alone in holding a position where his direct experience of being mentally ill fed into his new professional context. He spoke of how he negotiated these blurred boundaries between himself as 'service user', himself as artist, and himself as professional:

> *Now I work with mental health patients, I can't hide myself away. Because you're like . . . a guardian while you're at work. You just are. I've got other responsibilities, I think. And that's all because of my art; it's given me this background to what I do . . . When I work at the Beta Gallery sometimes my own history helps other people understand theirs. We're not encouraged to talk about our own stuff but I think who better to talk about, and in the context of talking about your own stuff, help other people . . . you work alongside people, you help people and people help you back just because of the processes that are involved in it.*

Mabel, an artist in her fifties with a long history of mental illness who also now works in community arts, echoed this dual role of helping and being helped, with both processes feeding into one's art practice and artistic identity:

> *Well I think being involved with other people who are also interested in the arts and also wanting to pursue art has really helped me because it's also given me a community where I can also exist and be amongst people. So part of being involved in the Arts Hub is having other people to share that process, to learn from each other.*

'Community arts' will for me always have 1980s undertones of draughty, poorly equipped spaces, cups of tea on Formica surfaces, murals and the almost bygone whiff of cigarette smoke. My own nostalgia and wariness came and went in waves while I heard stories which sometimes chimed with these memories – but invariably presented newer, more commercially savvy and strategically organized endeavours. Many of the people I spoke to expressed an allegiance to, and affection for, the projects and venues which had become the centre of their 'community arts practice'. In varying greatly, community arts projects nevertheless seemed to hold more similarities than differences. The predominant similarity was that of ethos – with a strong identification with Freirean concepts of equality, participation, and the value of experiential knowledge. A few spoke of community arts as being a medium for social and political change, and emerging in the narratives was the neo-liberal language suggestive of New Labour and the later Coalition government's discourse of social inclusion and volunteerism. There was also recognition of the attempt in community arts to balance the individual with the collective – a highly valued, yet admittedly tricky exercise. Whilst community art is often seen as fostering collaborative art and engagement, most of the people with whom I spoke focused mainly on 'their' art practice and interests. Even if artists had participated in joint ventures, it was their (solo) journey through this they chose to speak about. One reason for this may lie in a still closely held belief in the individualism of artistic practice and creativity, touched on in Chapter 2. While critiques and attempts to upturn this approach to thinking about creativity abound both in psychology (Glaveanu, 2010) and within the arts, as I turn to later on in this chapter, the artistic process as being an individual journey remains a dominant message of Western twenty-first-century discourse, despite attempts to reframe the artist as 'post-Cartesian' and replace the first person singular with the collaboration of first person plural (Roberts, 2007).

A further reason for the narratives of solo journeying may well lie in the design of the research recruitment through which these narratives were generated. In this we did not target and request the participation of groups of artists with mental health difficulties, but individuals. Another explanation may well lie in the personal and artistic journey many of the artists described, which I return to in Chapter 4 – a journey which involved an almost involuntary period of highly personal reflection, self-analysis and autobiographic encounter; a being alone with one's story – even in the company of others.

For many people involved in community arts who had been through the psychiatric gulag, the space to 'be' as a person that was provided by the community arts project and venue was highly prized. The sense of community amongst participants, as also found by Howells and Zelnik (2009), facilitated the formation of identity and provided a bridge to the wider community, and, as reported by Parr (2006: 151), community 'arts for mental health' projects 'involve relational geographies that assist people in creating senses of stability and belonging'. This was especially the case if it was nestled within a grassroots, largely non-hierarchical association of 'survivors' joined by the common interest of art. This offered a valued contrast to their life chapters within mental health services. There, they had always been positioned as patient, user, survivor or client in an asymmetrical relationship with doctors, psychiatrists and therapists. There, hierarchy was felt to be sedimented, stretching from sane and clinical, downwards. Fellow patients were joined not by a common thread of art, creativity, love of colour, texture, shape and form and expression – but by the common thread of illness and deficit.

Community art, including some innovative Arts in Health work in particular, was invariably held to be a vehicle away from this. This vehicle made sense – because it wasn't about the past, about the illness; it was about the now and the moving forward, about creating, meeting, talking, and re-configuring your story.

Andrew is a young, intense artist who had been diagnosed with schizophrenia in his early twenties. He spoke about how delicate the process of re-entering a social world was after spending time not only in hospitals and in the stultifying parallel reality of strong medication, but in a world of your own, into which, for a period of time, retreat had been total. Here is Andrew:

> . . . *the things that stop you from reintegrating into society are seemingly small . . . but if you had a break away from life, your community, your family or whatever, getting back to how things were is never going to be the same. That tiny little thing . . . It's a social thing. You've been with people all your life. You've never had a break away with them. I've had to rebuild that. I've lost something really small that keeps you as a social being. Being able to perceive other people's existence is quite difficult.*
>
> *But take another environment, like I go to nightclubs, and I can be pretty sure I'm not on a wavelength with most other people there. I think that people in that environment, they're lucky to share their experiences. They see themselves as on a level with everyone around them, even though they could be experiencing all kinds of different things. It's that tiny little thing of being part of a community which I think I lost when I got ill . . . again, it's very difficult to explain. I suppose that's rehabilitation.*

Community arts projects offered just the transitional place and space for this 'tiny little thing' to be enabled. Often positioned as free from the constraints of contemporary art fashions, clinical interpretations (see also Parr, 2006) and psychiatric diagnostic procedures, they commonly offered a studio culture with like-minded peers, and the possibility of a further stage (in both meanings of the word) of and for displaying and disclosing. This important but potentially risky act is one to which I return in Chapter 6, as it has particular ramifications for both the artist and the service user.

There can be little doubt that community arts and allied work such as Arts in Health initiatives play a vital role in the recovery journey of many people. People spoke of being 'saved' by such ventures, or of individuals finding themselves, others with whom to more authentically connect, or, indeed, a purpose. Some of these people had always done some form of art, or had lost it and found it again, through the chameleonic experience of mental illness. Others had been brought to art for the first time through involvement in an arts project targeted at service users, or through an element of serendipity where one simple idea on the part of a health worker provides a pivotal moment.

Mink is a 52-year-old woman who has a diagnosis of Dissociative Identity Disorder (DID), formerly known as multiple personality disorder. She has now used art over many years to achieve a level of insight into her identities formerly inaccessible through other therapies. She is also a practising artist who has had a number of solo exhibitions. She described how this journey began with a chance encounter with art:

> *In 2004, I had a support worker who suggested to me that we do some painting . . . we, when I say 'we', me and the other personalities . . . at that point there was seven of us . . . we started just painting on the back of wallpaper with my daughter's paints, we'd never painted before that, so after we'd been doing that for about three or four months, she said that*

she felt we should take our work more seriously and so I went and got some canvases and some acrylics and I haven't stopped painting . . .

Nuala, a photographer in her thirties whose story is stamped by the marks of both cancer and mental illness, also spoke of one such encounter:

I'm from Dublin. I kind of grew up in a pretty awful place, very violent alcoholic family, so that caused me to have depression from a very early age. As a kid I didn't have any interests, I didn't have any involvement with any kind of creative, or artistic thing, or anything really. I feel I was sort of crippled a lot by the way I grew up . . . I went into a therapeutic community and it was there that . . . it was located inside a hospital and one weekend when we had nothing to do the nurses bought us all some disposable cameras and took us out for a walk and got us taking photos and that was my very first of that kind of thing and I just loved it. With a camera I could just look through the viewfinder and with the few seconds I was looking through the viewfinder I could concentrate. I just needed a couple of seconds and I found that in just a couple of seconds I could actually do something. And it was wonderful . . . and that was my first introduction into it and I loved it straight away. It's [art's] been a massive part of my recovery although I wouldn't say I'm totally cured yet, not by a long shot.

For others still, it had been their illness itself, with its ways of both silencing you and yet demanding to be storied, which had brought them to seek a means of expression, and some instances of this are looked at in the next chapter.

Despite both community arts and projects which offered arts within the health system performing a vital role in people's recovery journey, there was invariably a sense of these projects, venues and initiatives being *temporary*. They were often based on short-term funding, the huge dedication of a few, a wing and a prayer and limited future planning. For some artists who were likely to use and even need the community project for a long time to come, this transitory feeling often added to an anxious, unsteady state of being. Those who used community arts as a stepping stone lamented the possible erasure of a service which had given them so much. François Matarasso, speaking of participatory arts projects, rather than community arts *per se*, notes the risk and impact of projects ending suddenly:

An abrupt withdrawal of creative opportunities, even if known about long in advance, may leave participants with little to do and wondering whether others placed the same value on the project as they did themselves. At worst, people may feel they have been lied to or used, and that the promises and new opportunities spoken about have been withdrawn.

(2013: 10)

A handful of artists alluded in their interviews to the political tensions of community art and its status, and expressed frustrations about its perceived 'low quality' aesthetic. It is worth taking some time here to describe the structural landscape in which this perception is nestled.

There is now a body of literature convincing in its claim that 'art works' for people with a range of health issues. Matarasso's oft-cited 1997 *Use or Ornament? The Social Impact of Participation in the Arts* found that the arts are essential to communities and have positive effects on people's wellbeing. Although heavily criticized by, amongst others, Merli (2002), Matarasso's research has played an important role in establishing a near-consensus in Britain among cultural policy makers. As briefly mentioned, however, this appropriation of the language of community arts engagement by the establishment has had an impact on the way in which we frame community and activism, and the ways in which we position the individual and the collective.

Hand in hand with this established turn to the arts for health has come pressure for researchers to develop a metric for measuring the benefits of arts programmes for the mentally ill, congruent with an Evidence Based Medicine (EBM) model. This positivistic approach to arts projects that take place within health settings places an obligation on Arts in Health to conform to a clinical standard of evaluation, and may be reproducing a now familiar 'what gets measured gets delivered' effect and contributing to a neglect of the non-market value of arts activity. As the link between arts and wellbeing has become embedded in policy discourse, critics have pointed out how this embrace can also be seen to be less about nurturing people's creativity and wellbeing and more about 'ham-fisted social engineering' (Kester, 2012). 'Inclusion' practices are thus seen as acting to mask social inequality rather than openly confront it (Bishop, 2006). As pointed out by Merli:

> making deprivation more acceptable is a tool to endlessly reproduce it. Social deprivation and exclusion arguably can be removed only by fighting the structural conditions which cause them. Such conditions will not be removed by benevolent arts programmes.
>
> (2002: 109)

Kwon (2002), too, has pointed out that community art projects can overlook the cultural and economic forces that render communities impoverished. In addressing the plight of the individual, we lose the potential for such projects to act on a larger and more complex scale, as transformative. Kwon is acerbic in her analysis that community arts may have a tendency to become patronizing and almost colonial, with 'well intentioned gestures for democratization', objectifying 'otherness' out of a 'lust for authentic histories and identities' (2002: 139). Love also takes issue with the reification of difference:

> it's one thing to encourage someone to find their 'own voice' and make work about their 'own experience,' but what if such an appeal to this so-called unerring veracity only serves to keep that person in their 'own place'; to fix or reify that voice or experience as essentially and irrevocably marginal and different?
>
> (2005: 161)

Yet amidst the astute political objections and ideological battles there can be little doubt that community arts have acted, and continue to act in the lives of many, to raise awareness and galvanize. Darrell, the painter we met earlier, spoke of battling his own history and finding a way to make sense of it, his diagnosis and the role of his art specifically through his involvement with a community arts group with whom he now works. It is a group that is dedicated to working with people with Borderline Personality Disorder:

> *I suppose I got into it [art] through getting involved in an organization. There's a thing called Personality People which aimed to raise awareness of personality disorders through artwork. I wanted to be able to give the likes of myself and guys on the street access to art and materials and be able to express themselves. There's a lot of artwork and artists out there that never get into the mainstream of art because they are considered to be outsiders, or they're in the margins. I think trying to break through the barriers that way, with organizations . . . is the way . . .*

Community projects were described as having raised awareness of mental health; of the arts world; of possible routes into education; of routes to resistance; and crucially providing a link to a group of like-minded peers. But part of the difficulty in critiquing work which continues under the rubric of community arts or Arts in Health is that while indeed such practice varies greatly in the degree to which it is collaborative and the degree to which it contributes to wider political engagement and resistance, and while it arguably does function as a bandage on a deeply injured social order and acts to sequester resistance into a space in which it can do no harm or disrupt the status of community art in the shadow of high art – still on a *micro* level, community arts practice, and Arts in Health initiatives, can, and do, act as a vital catalyst for change for some individuals. A few artists described the intricacies of a journey which began with the powerlessness of deep illness, travelled through art as personal expression, and on into the role of activist and informed expert by experience. They were armed with a formidable array of artistic and intellectual tools with which to interrogate an art system they viewed as fundamentally flawed, unequal and elitist – and they were on the move still.

Transition: swimming upstream into the mainstream

If, or when, community arts in any of its manifestations no longer served the developing artistic persona, some interviews described a point experienced as a lull, or a vacuum. When this space became uncomfortable some returned to their known project or place even though they felt they had 'grown out of it' as artists and individuals. Others started their own community group, or roused further engagement amongst like-minded peers and provided offshoot projects. For some, a slow road into further and higher education in the arts now began. Fatima, a Turkish painter in her forties, was one:

> *So I started painting. I went to Painters Cafe and Jane there taught me to use colours, to draw and then . . . I went to St Michael's and there was free materials which . . . and at*

that time I was really poor so I used the free materials to draw copies of Chagall, Picasso, Van Gogh, you name it I drew it. And then I thought sod it . . . I thought I'm not going to do the same as when I was a sheep, I'm going to study. So I went and did my GNVQ . . . and then I went and did my Foundation and then in 2003 I started my first degree. So I finished university, I got a 2:1. Then in 2006 I got accepted for the Masters . . .

Fatima's characteristically flippant description belies the difficulty of the task of getting into, let alone through, education while continuing to battle mental illness. For those who took this road, it was one rarely spoken of as being easy, dotted as it was with breakdowns, relapses, periods of disruption through changed medication, bouts of depression, psychotic attacks, deep self-doubt and self-persecution – not to mention the sheer cost, prohibitive to most. Sometimes the decision and determination made people sail close to the wind:

In the summer before I started at university I had . . . I was admitted again [into hospital]. I was discharged from the hospital on, I think it was Monday afternoon . . . and I went and started at the college on the Wednesday.

(Pippa)

I enrolled – didn't have a clue about whether I'd be able to get through the first term let alone the course . . . I changed my meds, just before, was feeling sick and queasy. But I felt like I was on a roll, there was an idea that I had to follow . . . I wanted it [art college] so bad . . .

(Thomas)

In earlier research I carried out with art students who have histories of mental illness (Sagan, 2009b), interviewees spoke of the tricky terrain of negotiating the pressures, stigma, cost and demands of higher education. This route was by no means smooth, yet there were many stories of education playing a life-affirming and transformative role. Student stories also described the enhanced systems of support enabled by the UK Widening Participation initiative linked to the Labour government of 1997–2010. The narratives of those who entered higher education frequently referred to the hard work of some of Widening Participation's foot soldiers – the mental health teams, personal tutors who went the extra mile, and experienced university and college counsellors. They spoke appreciatively of flexible and sensitive systems which allowed for the interruptions of study due to ill health, and the sheer exhilaration, finally, of being in an arts environment where an identity as mental health user was far subordinate to one of artist and student. The descriptions of being in higher arts education spoke of the boosted efforts of the arts institution at making community links through participatory outreach work. Bizarrely, sometimes these initiatives returned people with whom I spoke to their community and mental health roots within a participatory project between the institution and a local community – an irony not lost on the student.

Whether people went on to education, other arts projects, or carried on working at their art practice from within sheltered accommodation or other sometimes unsuitable home environments, what stamped their narratives was the emergence of an *artistic identity*. This artistic identity appeared to be crucial in the agentic reconfiguration that people undertook of themselves – from service user to *other*:

> . . . *when you start to exhibit you change your label from service user or person with a personality disorder to artist and that's a much more holistic, a much happier title and it's also something that makes me feel like a complete person.*

(Crystal)

Both in the art work itself and in the narratives, individuals appeared to engage in what Ricoeur (1970) calls 'progressive and regressive hermeneutics', a parallel exploration of one's history, *and* a shedding of old skins. This process of identity reconfiguration had several stages, and will be looked at in more detail in the next chapter. In a journey which sometimes ran from, or indeed back into and again out of, art therapy/Arts in Health, to community arts, to arts education, there were 'hybrid' professionals met with along the way. These roles – as art project worker, artist educator, arts health practitioner, mental health artist, non-therapy-oriented artist – were often, but not always, occupied by people who had themselves experienced some form of mental illness. Some of the tensions of these roles are described well by Langley Brown (2012), and they emerge in people's narratives of transition. They serve to remind us, as Broderick (2011: 95) states, that 'The specific subject domains of "arts" and "health" do not exist as concrete entities, but are shifting, amorphous and contested, subject to competing knowledge claims within their own disciplines.'

There were many stages of transition that people spoke of in the journey of their arts practice. The journey was by no means always linear, and never smooth. One stage which individuals often struggled, it seemed, to articulate was that from being an artist connected to community arts, Arts in Health work, 'Outsider Arts' galleries and venues that specifically promoted the art of the mentally ill, to one of an artist *not* connected with these places and categories. This deliberate, gradual repositioning was articulated in various ways, but these sometimes opaque pieces of narrative held the indecision, self-analysis and frustration of this process as well as experimentations with the limitations of words and terminology. As Marty put it, '*I'm an artist that happens to have mental health problems; I'm not a mental health artist.*'

And here is Leonne:

> *I'm not a 'mental health artist' [makes scare marks]. I'm not an 'outsider artist'. In fact I'm more of an insider artist as everything I create is about what is happening inside – me . . . Just because I'm bipolar doesn't mean I have to stay in community arts or work with others who have a mental health condition, but it's like . . . I'm not interesting unless I'm a 'Bipolar Artist' so I can't escape that . . . that label, again . . .*

In writing from an Australian mental health and art context, Gwinner and colleagues described similar issues. They observed that artists with mental health difficulties, once known as 'outsiders', were:

highly likely to find it difficult to move outside that category if their mental health issues are known, even when their art itself is not a product or a referent to their mental state. Thus an artist with a mental illness is inhibited from moving away from the health context into the wider art community.

(Gwinner *et al.*, 2010: 30)

So trying to escape labelling appears to continue for the mentally ill artist, entailing trying on different artistic identities. Lyle Rexer (2005) in writing about Outsider Art cautions that while the term has the potential to add positive value to the artist's work, it can, by the same token, imprison; and Gwinner and colleagues (2010: 34) also highlight the bind of a 'visual psychopathology'.

In some ways, for the people with whom I spoke, this quest to move beyond the prison of a label had become *the* quest. Much as coming to terms with being 'mad' (a term some people had a considered preference for), a 'survivor', a 'service user' or someone with 'mental health difficulties' had taken time and a wrestling with discourse, so now positioning oneself as an artist, Outsider or not, was a crucial but no straightforward act. A growing awareness of oneself and a developing vision of one's art led to an inevitable confrontation with structural forces at play. These enabled or disabled art production, invited or hindered exhibition, encouraged or discouraged engagement. They also determined 'quality' in the art work.

My art practice is really limited for a number of reasons. There are obstacles that get in the way of it. Partly the fatigue itself is an obstacle, and the poverty that goes with that, in terms of getting access to resources to pursue my interest in the arts. I used to be able to – back in the past when you could get access to community education, courses and things – I used to go on a lot of courses, get involved in studying so I could get access to resources. Nowadays even those courses are beyond my means. I can't afford them. So my art practice is very limited.

(Paul)

At the time of writing it is still too early to say what the impact will be of the introduction in England of personal budgets fully implemented by the Coalition government by April 2013, and whether new opportunities for funding (Hebron and Taylor, 2012) will materialize. What is clear is that mental ill health is frequently accompanied and exacerbated by financial hardship. Economic constraints on one's art practice, however small and humble that practice may be, were spoken of frequently, as were the interruptions and irruptions of ill health. But there were other related, yet less obvious barriers encountered to the development of an art practice. Mink, the artist we met earlier, diagnosed with DID, who paints as a number of personalities, describes herself (themselves) as 'untrained' artists. She describes trying to swim in the 'mainstream' rather than 'outsider' art world and alludes to the 'cultural capital' gained through going through art education:

I've tried to get out of it [mental health-related art world], desperately . . . and it's a struggle . . . I showed my work to a gallery, I was pleased that they liked the work . . . I didn't know anything, at that point about Outsider Art and I didn't know how cliquey the art world was . . . and so, (sighs) you know, I think I can take a couple of the personalities and say they fit better into the category of Outsider Art . . . but . . . (sighs) what I'm finding now I'm up against . . . in the beginning, I entered for competitions . . . um . . . exhibitions, I got into a few . . . that was really exciting . . . and I go in for things thinking I won't say about the DID because I think that's the best idea, but with the Outsider Art I tend to get in more . . . but what I'm finding now is . . . I thought Outsider Art was . . . it's some battle . . . was more or less for untrained artists, but it's not, so now what I'm up against is trained artists, they may have had a breakdown, been in hospital for a week and are now classing themselves as an Outsider . . . and so now, what I find unfair is I'm classed as an Outsider Artist and the ordinary galleries are not really interested and yet the artists that have been trained can go in on both sides if they've had a psychiatric problem or been an inpatient somewhere . . . I just think it's getting tougher 'cause you're up against trained artists even to get into Outsider Art exhibitions now . . . and some of them . . . well, they're really good artists and (pause) . . . yeah . . . they know a lot more, they're more experienced about everything, they know how to get in to galleries . . . I mean I haven't got any arty friends, my friends have always been psychiatric patients . . . I haven't got any friends in the art world, whereas when you've been trained, you've gone through the college, all your friends tend to be artists as well, you can have group exhibitions together, you know the art world and you know how it is, but you've got the other side, you can go into Outsider Art . . . think it's quite unfair . . .

Artists' narratives questioned the degree to which 'Outsider Art' was a helpful category, even though, for some, it had offered opportunities for establishing a genre and gaining exposure. Now an established and lucrative industry, with dealers and curators cultivating the myth of 'outsiderness' in order to pump-prime sales, artist and art therapist David Maclagan[4] observes:

> Outsider art has now been around for about sixty years, Dubuffet started his collection in 1947 . . . during that time, exhibitions, catalogues, magazines, galleries and so on that deal in Outsider Art have proliferated . . . it's part of the curriculum in art colleges and art schools . . . once upon a time Outsider Art was as it were 'out there' and entirely separate and uncontaminated by mainstream culture and now it has become, in a number of ways incorporated . . .

Some artists nevertheless remained unperturbed by these categories and denied that they presented barriers or challenges. Some of these were individuals who had reached a point in their practice with which they felt content, for a number of personal reasons, variably articulated. They were not aspiring in terms of wanting more, bigger and better exposure or connection with the mainstream art world. For some, an everyday, modest practice, which they used as part of a strategy to maintain balance and wellbeing, was gift and arrival enough. As Vita, a 65-year-old ceramic artist who relished at long last being able to acquire her own studio space put it:

It [art] gives a purpose and meaning to the day and a sense of achievement . . . and it's really thrilling when someone likes a piece so much they buy it!

For others, however, there was an earnest quest underway for a future as an artist with the prospect of more opportunity to enter stimulating arenas, projects and collaborations. For these, the terrain was bumpy with ideological potholes, and busy with new discourses with which many felt less than fluent.

Transition: a place to be

Crystal, a vocal and charismatic social artist, tussled with strong allegiances to community, the working class and those with mental ill health while having a passion and energetic commitment to the development of her practice:

Phee [university mentor] was telling me that community practice and fine art gallery practice are almost at absolutely opposite ends of the spectrum and I need to think about where I want to position myself . . . so in that point of view, I thought I didn't want to do community stuff. But also I mentioned to you in an earlier interview about this overwhelming need to give back what's been given to me . . .

Liz Atkin, establishing herself as an artist working with her own body/illness, feels the pull of a more 'highbrow' place for her art, but grounds herself in communities:

. . . this hasn't been about Art with a big A . . . I exist in [that] community space . . . I think working with communities of people is far more powerful and important for me, ethically . . . I'm not looking for a 'big thing' – I haven't come to this through 'fine art', I didn't train as an artist, I haven't studied painting, I studied theatre and dance. I use a camera but I'm not trained as a photographer, I have a range of experience that led me to this practice anyway so it feels a bit fake for me to align myself more with highbrow art world stuff, because I don't know it . . . I don't come from it, I'm not aiming for it as a kind of elite form . . .

Many of the artists with whom I spoke had made a patchwork journey through the mental health system and whatever arts projects and art therapy were available therein, into higher arts education and thereby into what was felt to be a new sociocultural order. In presenting the journey as one of transition and linearity, it is all too easy to suggest this process is smooth. It is not; either in terms of the individual's positioning, re-positioning and identity transformations, or in terms of the significant structural barriers which continue to bar access to welfare, to education and to a cultural milieu still predominantly based on privilege. In challenging such barriers, over and again, and finally identifying her practice as one of a social artist, Crystal had arrived at a place where she was a full-time social artist, keeping a strong allegiance to her roots within a lower socioeconomic grouping which had experienced added marginalization and hardship as a result of mental illness. By entering an identity as a social artist and beginning to navigate the 'Art World', Crystal and others like her were embracing an artist identity within an expanding, but heavily contested field of 'relational practices' which have burgeoned in the art world since the early 1990s and held an allure for those with strong community roots.

Coined by the French curator Nicolas Bourriaud who arguably made an existing set of socially engaged practices more art-market-ready simply by the creation of a marketable title, the term 'Relational Aesthetics' describes a wide range of art practices. These take as their subject human relations and the social context in which such relations arise, rendering the artist's voice 'subordinate to the forces of reproducibility and general social technique' (Roberts, 2007: 115). Such practices hold out appealing possibilities for bringing together the lived experiences of marginalization, a social conscience and a commitment to partici-patory ventures. They also raise important questions about the meaning and purpose of art in society and about the role of the artist and the experience of the audience as participant. There are resonances in the genre and its debates for artists who have encountered the binary subject positions of doctor/patient, insider/outsider, sane/insane, and expressions of otherness in the designated role they have fought in those relationships. They may already have grappled with questions widespread in relational art practice of the gaze and objectification, of who is watching who, and who has the power to represent and to interpret. Relational practices, in working the nebulous liminal areas neither gallery nor hospital, may also offer the experience of 'potential space' (Winnicott, 1971), one that is safe but playful, and provide a point where the inner world of the artist can make more risky connections with the outer world.

Some of the artists with whom I spoke had a take on their work which suggested they positioned it as *dialogic* but not 'relational' or 'participatory' as these contested terms have largely come to be defined. They expressed a developing artistic persona and ideology more in line with the Bakhtinian concept of 'dialogism' in which their art is a response to what has been before, and in anticipation of connection with a spectator, or consumer, who, in turn, will respond:

> *I do look [at Outsider Art] and try and push it further, through my work, so it's more confrontational . . . I think the audience expects a certain thing of the . . . the mentally ill in art and I want to turn that on its head. But also . . . to inform and yeah . . . educate – and then work back the responses to that into my work . . .*

> (Laurence)

The work is not seen as produced in a vacuum but rather as part of a dynamic process, describing and re-describing, sharing language, ideas, motifs – there is also, of course, an often referred to continuing dialogue, between the illness and the art, to which I will come back in Chapters 4 and 5. Grant Kester (2004: 10) argues that dialogical art aims to 'replace the "banking" style of art in which the artist deposits an expressive content into a physical object, to be withdrawn later by the viewer, with a process of dialogue and collaboration'. Interviewee Liz Atkin, while producing images of herself, and working largely as an individual artist, nevertheless speaks of the interaction and dialogue with other artists, patients whom she meets through a hospital collaboration, and the public and residents of the area in which she lives with a community of artists, all as being an essential part of her work, feeding into such a process:

> *I do collaborate with other artists which has been a really fantastic new venture for me . . . and also it's been a big thing in terms of trust, because I've had to trust people being with my body, and trust that encounter which was difficult for me when I was ill . . . I've also met patients now, who are being treated for the same illness . . . who are at a different stage in their experience and it's been good for me to meet others and share . . . some of my hope of being better . . .*

> *I live in a community of artists and we regularly have open studios . . . the public literally come to my house (laughs) and walk around and you know, you have a very direct encounter with people meeting the art works for the first time and asking questions . . . it opens up a dialogue which is useful.*

While relational practices which espouse collaboration and participation enjoy current popularity, they are not new. Claire Bishop argues that rather than representing a 'new' development, this 'social turn' is part of 'an ongoing history of attempts to rethink art collectively' (2012: 3). She links its more recent manifestation to the fall of communism, reverberations of which arguably deprived 'the left of the last vestiges of the revolution that had once linked political and aesthetic radicalism' (Bishop, 2006: 178).

Relational practices are based on a belief that by encouraging an audience to join in, the artist can promote new emancipatory social relations and unseat social orders – aspirations which echo the community arts and grassroots seeds of many artists working in this area, or their political aspirations. The artist Ana Laura López de la Torre, for example, recognizes that her work has evolved from political and experimental art of the 1960s and 1970s, and describes her model of practice as one in which the artist has a long-term commitment and declared investment in the communities within which they work. She maintains that:

> For me, the whole gist of working in community is simply an extension of how I live my life, I do art in my community with others, the same way that I live in community with others, I believe that the best life is one shared.
>
> (López de la Torre, 2013)

But not all relational or social practice is born in a specific location with a commitment to the place and its people; neither is it all aligned with political or social change. The status of collaborators/audience/participants in socially engaged art work varies widely, with authorial balance hotly debated. Such practices operate within the world of contemporary 'high' art discourse and are even frequently undertaken by artists whose work also functions within the art market. This point has particular poignancy for artists who have arrived in this milieu through a journey which shares characteristics with those journeys described earlier, and who have perhaps, *en route*, been positioned or positioned themselves as belonging to the poorly defined genre of 'Outsider Art'. For it is one thing to come from a relatively conventional background as an artist, to enjoy the privilege and understand its discourse, and to then *elect* to position yourself as a social or relational artist, taking up the mantra of participation and playing the risk area of 'High Art v. Community Art'. It is quite another to come from the 'outside', of art, of society, or indeed 'sanity'; to experience stigma and exclusion; to then move at some personal cost towards professional or semi-professional practice, and *then* to work within an area which aims to be located again on a porous border between high art and community art. One of the many ironies in this positioning and repositioning dance is that participatory art has been accused of objectifying 'otherness' while 'otherness' is felt to be the very watermark of the artist with a background of mental illness.

There remains the question of whether such artists, involved in participatory, social or relational art, overturn the conventional idea of artist with which many of the participants tussled as part of their identity reconfiguring. Kester (2004: 171), again, is sceptical. For him, community-based work 'created' by artists serves to reinforce a view of a given 'disadvantaged' community or constituency as an instrumentalized and fictively monolithic entity to be 'serviced by the visiting artist'. Elsewhere, Kester (1995: x) also criticizes artists who 'imagine that they can transcend the very real differences that exist between themselves and a given community by a well-meaning rhetoric of aesthetic "empowerment"'. Beech (2008), meanwhile, argues that the practice of relational art merely extends the commodification of art, through incorporating social events into the range of art commodities, questioning again whether any disruption is occurring in the status quo.

So to what extent these artists' practices offer an alternative way of envisioning art works and their production is the subject of some debate. To approach the question we need to consider the status of High Art and what, for purposes of expedience, I bunch under the umbrella term 'Community Art', inadequate as this term is to properly address the very many different practices and ideologies within this category. And we must also be aware that the contested term 'community' is one which, having gone through the contortions of neo-liberalization and become co-opted into Big Society rhetoric, one 'big in heart though short of state funding' (Sennett, 2012: 250), is virtually meaningless. Yet the idea, or image, of community art figures prominently in the narratives of artists with whom I spoke, and clearly serves a particular function in their experience, imaginings and aspirations.

There is, without doubt, work produced in a space which straddles the worlds of health and High Art which offers insights into the nature of mental illness; one thinks of the work of Aidan Shingler, for example, whose work has explored the experience of schizophrenia, or that of Bobby Baker and her journey through the psychiatric system; the Japanese artist Yayoi Kusama, now in her eighties and still working from within the walls of a psychiatric institution yet exhibiting at prestigious mainstream galleries; and Shona Illingworth, offering multidisciplinary works which investigate memory and invite public engagement. Through their undisputedly powerful work the audience can learn about other people's experience of illness; of disjuncture; or recognize aspects of their own experience in ways poignant, disturbing, even beautiful. Yet there remains an unshakable order in the (art) world and some resilient realities impenetrable to many. Chloe Shalini spoke candidly of '*the pointless garden paths*' you walk up trying to get into galleries:

> . . . *the way the art world works is that it helps if you've gone to college . . . it's dominated by people who have already got a status of being known, who have been through a final show at college at least . . .*

Within a given socioeconomic order, art institutions, and routes to them either as spectator or creator (or both), remain largely static. While the space, connectivity and dissemination properties of the internet have certainly eroded the hold of some hierarchical and elite practices (but Bishop (2012: 190) usefully raises the question of 'the difference between a work of art and social networking'), there are no more 'alternative' spaces or practices now than in the 1960s. Artists such as Shingler, Baker, Kusama, Bourgeois, and Illingworth do, in different ways, ripple the surface of the debate now and then and give the audience a valuable and different angle on a subject. But opposition, resistance and debate are an integral part of the ideological composition under capitalism. As Grayson Perry quipped in his third Reith Lecture for Radio 4 in 2013:

> And the creative rebel – they like to think they're sticking it to the man, they're sticking it to the capitalist system . . . But of course what they don't realise – by being all inventive and creative, they're actually playing into capitalism's hands because the lifeblood of capitalism is new ideas. They need new stuff to sell!

But art, inherently limited in ability to challenge hegemony, has always done precisely this, its renegade quality quickly becoming subsumed into the conventional art machine. Once such work is appropriated into the relatively static infrastructure of the art world, any act of dissent in the work is immediately diluted.

Andrew Locke, whose current work explores the dark hinterlands of mental illness, dance trance and drugs, had no illusions about his art, or that of others coming from within mental health services, as ultimately occupying a subversive space or performing a more provocative role in the social order:

> *I think the modernist breakdown in the twentieth century has facilitated a lot of exposure to artists who are outside of the art world and doing interesting things. But of course, it gets absorbed by the art world . . . when there's an exhibition.*

The relentlessness of that absorption was revealed through the removal, in 2013, of a Banksy painting depicting child labour from a wall in Haringey, in north London, and its rapid re-emergence in an auction in Miami. After local protests were widely reported, the Miami auction house announced withdrawal of the piece from sale, and Haringey Council Leader Claire Kober credited the community campaigning with being instrumental in this. But we should be cautious of seeing this event as a victory for the community, or for the place of graffiti as the people's art, let alone a victory for the expression of the anti-global capitalist message of the graffiti piece. The event demonstrated, rather, the elasticity and rapidity with which Art Capitalism deftly embraces all as consumer item, and the ways in which protest and media coverage of it serve to add monetary value to a well-stocked art warehouse – all part of living through what Grayson Perry, in his earlier mentioned Reith Lecture, referred to as 'the end state of art'. The very language of resistance itself, the lingua franca of avant-garde artists, has been appropriated and neutered:

> We find curators, educational programmers, and gallery directors expressing their desire for 'disrupting notions of subject,' 'disturbing notions of demographics,' and 'disrupting regimes of representation.' Others worry about how to 'challenge' viewers or provide them with 'difficult experiences'. In part this can be ascribed to the gradual migration, over the past decade or so, of language traditionally associated with the artistic personality into the professional rhetoric of curators and programmers.
>
> (Kester, 2012)

If the domains of community art and high art remain rigid in a status quo, then what, if any, *mobility* is possible between these domains? Questioning this mobility, and the structures and systems which support or hinder it, remains crucial. Not only because the narratives of artists and artists-becoming directly addressed it, but because it is impossible to extricate art practice, and our aspirations or angers about it, from the prevailing social structures. Bourdieu (1993) gave us useful terms and tools with which to analyse how working-class people are excluded from appreciation of art by their lack of familiarity with the requisite aesthetic codes. He spoke of how 'habitus' – our 'feel for the game' – the result of a long process of inculcation which begins in childhood, endows some with an entry point into culture while denying others, and how cultural capital, an internalized code or cognitive acquisition, equips some with an almost 'innate' competence for deciphering cultural relations and artefacts. His analysis makes blatant the power relations in social life. Kester, again, states that Bourdieu's analysis urges us to

> question the tendency of some community artists to unproblematically identify their interests (professional, political, creative, moral, economic, etc.) with those of the community. Too often community artists imagine that the very real differences that exist between themselves and a given community can be transcended by a well meaning rhetoric of aesthetic 'empowerment'.
>
> (Kester, 1995)

Such analysis and incisive critiques of the political and economic realities of the contemporary art world illuminate the stark divisions of the domains which flowed in and out of the narratives of artists with mental health difficulties. But Bourdieu's (1977) presentation of the ways that comportment and structures of taste, preference and desire reflect and reproduce societal hierarchies and positions is one which problematizes agency and dissent, and can foreclose on attempts to express either. Caught in the confluence of the competing and compelling discourses of high art, community and outsider art, service-user empowerment, self-help and an enduring language of artist as individual, the people I interviewed were making difficult choices about their identity, their art and their health – and battling the constraints on mobility from one domain to another. These domains, while being more porous than I may have depicted, do from time to time admit leakages and entertain troubled boundaries. And it is within such leakages and troubled boundaries that some artists do find a space conducive to working productively. Such a space may be thought of as 'smooth', using Deleuze and Guattari's (Deleuze *et al.*, 2011) conceptualization, where space, allowing growth and dynamic transformation, functions as an alternative to the hierarchical and confining areas characteristic of 'striated' space. In such a space, competing allegiances can play and both agency and dissent find expression.

Narratives of people who had been in and out of art therapy, in and out of projects loosely under the Arts and Health umbrella, and in and out of 'Community Arts' with its small galleries, collective studio space and café/atelier setting still spoke of a 'next step' which was invariably envisaged as entering higher education (still mainly referred to as 'art college') and/or setting up their own studio and website, thus beginning the long slog of self-promotion and juggling artistic pursuit with needing to earn money – in short, *what the traditional stereotype of the artist does*. And while this speaks of the rigidity of sociocultural structures and stratifications, on a micro level we must also question by what right do we disparage such aspirations to get onto what Grayson Perry called the 'fixed rung' of art college, when these aspirations are held by those from non-traditional backgrounds, from lower socioeconomic groups, or indeed the mental health system.

Notes

1 For a comprehensive overview of mental health history, readers are referred to the very useful timeline compilation of Andrew Roberts, a Middlesex University Resource, freely available at: http://studymore.org.uk/mhhtim.htm (accessed July 2014).

2 It is beyond the scope of this chapter to enter into current debates within art therapy regarding modality and nomenclature. Readers are referred, in the first instance, to the highly readable *Art Therapy* by Edwards (London: Sage, 2004); and *Healing Arts: The History of Art Therapy*, by Hogan (London: Jessica Kingsley, 2001).

3 The developing discipline of Arts in Health does not receive the attention it deserves here and readers are referred to Broderick (2011), Daykin and Byrne (2006) and Stickley (2012) for an oversight of the issues, context and research in the area.

4 *The View from Outside*, David Maclagan and Livy Powell. Video, Institute of Art and Ideas, available at http://iai.tv/video/the-view-from-outside (accessed September 2014).

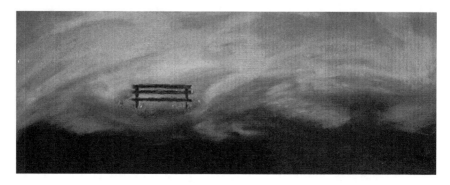

I will wait for you even in the middle of the night

4   Lost for words,
   found by image

Art celebrates with peculiar intensity the moments when the past reinforces
the present and in which the future is a quickening of what now is.
(John Dewey, 1934)

More than sixty people spoke to me about their illness, their wellness and their
art. Usually face to face but sometimes on the phone; one to one, in pairs, in
groups, in galleries, universities, cafés, community centres, hospitals and studios.
Sometimes we also spoke through extended email conversations, some of which
spanned years. I was humbled, time and again, by people's generosity with their
stories, their time, their open disclosures. Sometimes people told me that they
found the telling useful; it helped them to reflect on things, think things differently.
I was not a counsellor to them or a mental health professional or a friend. My ear
and I existed in the blurred and privileged zone of the researcher, and whilst I was
aware of the possible interplay of transference and countertransference and the
inherent problematics of an interview in which potentially the psychic traffic of
both interviewee and interviewer was travelling, my aim was not to pursue this line
of enquiry. It was, however, to draw on my therapeutic training only in so far as
it aided the establishment of a good listening relationship which might enable
the speaker to make freer connections with her experience and a more intimate
depiction of these.[1] In the best of cases, a space seemed to be opened up in the
telling and the listening, resonant of Winnicott's 'potential space', where
subjectivities played and intermingled. There was often a human warmth and a
pliable quality between us where stories deepened, slowed.

   Much has been written about 'first person narratives', 'illness narratives' and the
so-called 'urge to purge' by which, some say, these are precipitated. Sociologist
Mike Bury (2001: 265) has suggested that an emphasis on personal narratives is
part and parcel of late modernist cultures, where there is a 'loosening of the
authority of the "grand narratives" of science and medicine in the ordering of
everyday experience and especially in response to illness'. Professor of Psychology
Gail Hornstein in the US has compiled a comprehensive list of First Person
Narratives of people with mental illness, consisting of more than 700 titles,
testimony to the lengths to which people have gone to tell their story. Sociologist
Arthur Frank (1995) and psychiatrist and anthropologist Arthur Kleinman (1988)

amongst others have produced persuasive accounts of why illness will tell itself, and the forms that telling may take. Much of this genre is concerned with mental health and urges health professionals to value the stories that are collected in their profession. Proponents of storied approaches to working with people ask that they and others trying to better understand mental illness view the diagnostic categorization of the psychiatric interview as an unrepresentative slice of the person's autobiography, and one which can only go so far. They propose that first person stories of illness offer a counter narrative, a small but important stand confronting the tyranny of expert language (Harper, 2002) and the vast vocabularies of deficit (Gergen, 1990) through which the mentally ill person is portrayed.

Illness narratives are located within what has become known as the narrative turn, a well-documented move within the social sciences which takes as its starting point a fervent interest in people's stories, the way they are told and what function the telling holds. Such enquiry sometimes uneasily combines modern debates about individual human experience with postmodern concerns with language and agency. This turn is linked to a number of other social-scientific moves in the late twentieth and early twenty-first centuries: an increased interest in qualitative methods more generally, partly in response to the over-reliance on positivist methods and their authoritative control over research and the stories which are told within it *about* others rather than *by* them; and a turn to language, both spoken and written, triggering immediate questions about power and reflexivity in the exchanged word. A turn, too, to autobiography and the unconscious – an unconscious which ignites the telling of a life story and backdrops, perhaps, our apparently insatiable lust for these tellings. The gathering of stories, surely the oldest of methodologies for probing human experience, accompanies the turn, too, to collaborative, participant-centred research, often exploiting newly accessible audiovisual means of working with people and groups.

Some of these turns and focal points overlap each other and are reflected in popular imagery and text. The rash of disclosure in the 'Oprahfication' of TV; do-it-yourself videos documenting and displaying soul-searching; a new-found interest in genealogy, popularized through online family tree sites; blogs; Twitter. Myself in 140 characters. In 2013, the 'selfie' entered the *Oxford Dictionary*, so commonplace was the act of snapping a photo of our own good self on our own good smartphone. My Self, by My Self. Art too, as I described in the previous chapter, brushes shoulders with the popular appetite for autobiographic pursuit; participation and the social-scientific thirst for story, placing the overlooked into the position, perhaps, of over-watched.

Both narrative research and the deluge of first person disclosures and confessionals in popular media demand that we question who is being portrayed, by whom, and via what language. Postmodern perspectives argue that positioning 'the subject' as maintaining an essential core of self and identity, one amenable to revealing through language, is fundamentally flawed (Henriques *et al.*, 1998). The 'self' in these perspectives is contingent, not existing in the modern sense, let alone awaiting discovery, as in humanistic discourse. It is being made, rather, and unmade through different sociocultural contexts; the 'subject' one constituted by discursive practices. All of which renders any 'trust' in the transparency of the spoken word naïve – and as contributing to persisting myths about the 'individual' and the 'who' that I claim to 'be'.

These unsettling and profound perspectives have been challenged. Questions have been asked about where the extreme end of poststructuralist theory leaves us both in terms of the meaning making which is part of the human package, and reflexivity, which remains at the core of human agency and understanding. The heavy emphasis on language and context, too, has been charged with engulfing the person (Dunne, 1995), leaving no room for investigating what goes on *inside* people – what recourse to agency there is, and what forms resistance to the dominant culture may take. It leaves us, some have argued, with an unremitting pessimism and a scientific discourse that offers little emancipatory leverage.

The narratives in this book, like all narratives, were heard and read through a filter. This filter is one that acknowledges that while our identities are ascribed to us by the protean and fluid nature of cultural, social, economic, and political contexts, we are also shaped by our own *interpretations* and reactions to these, and through unconscious dynamics. The social and the psychic are hereby intertwined, and mutually constitutive. While our life stories are formed by discursive and sociocultural practices, there are 'eruptions' within these where we reconfigure, test out, reflect upon, reject or adopt the dominant narrative being spun out of our own mouths. The stories we construct, to make sense of our lives, as Dan McAdams (2008: 242) suggests, 'are fundamentally about our struggle to reconcile who we imagine we were, are, and might be . . .'.

Phenomenological approaches to narrative maintain that to reflect on our experience and to construct a story about ourselves, a sense of ownership is necessary – a sense of 'mineness' which provokes us to reject or to question the narrative threads which feel 'less than' mine, or alien to me in the making of a narrative identity. This concept of narrative identity provides a conceptual means by which the gulf separating an essentialist principle of selfhood on the one hand and the postmodern precept of the self as illusory on the other can be minimized. Psychoanalytic understandings of the person which accept unconscious dynamics as also being at play suggest that admittance of these provides for an even more complex picture of who/what we are. These two ideologies, far from being antithetical (Csordas, 2012; Good, 2012), may offer combined insights into ways of working with subjectivity, not as a product, but as a dynamic state.

In working with narratives I held these formulations of the person in mind and a non-essentialist view of identity. Taking an approach of respect and caution while looking at what may be revealed in people's stories about what needs are being met, how strategies are being deployed, and what resolutions, if any, are being indicated, there was also no certainty of interpretation. There was no adherence to the 'life story' as a true or enduring account, and indeed, in people's narratives the voices and words of others – of policy makers, care professionals, self-help gurus and popular psychologists – could be heard, as no doubt is the case with all our stories in which are embedded a collage of the voices of others.

But the narrator, however constituted, takes a moment by moment opportunity to reconfigure a story and minutely adjust 'narrative identity', to reflect to whatever degree possible, and to re-script her or his story. There was fidelity to the notion that through the telling, and re-configuring, some sense in which art was being used, understood and apprehended within this given life story, would breathe through. This forefronting of the micro of the person is also intentional; as it is through these instances of the micro that the macro of structures and systems that produce and delimit the mentally ill in society may be laid bare. So too are exposed the ways that people have sought to challenge these, one way being through their art practice.

So how does telling one's story have the positive effects reported by some of the participants in this research? It may be that providing a testimony, a first person narrative, offers a means by which some feel they are counterbalancing, in however small a way, the weight of narrative *about* people, with narrative *by* them. This is especially salient for those who spoke with me who had been through the de-voicing and discourse-colonization of the 'psychiatric gulag' (Hartill, 1998). Or it could be that the narrative interview, where one is being listened to and being heard, uninterrupted and respected, itself has a restorative impact (Frosh, 2002). At the heart of both possibilities is the notion of a storied self, a view that human psychology has a narrative form and that we think, perceive, behave, feel and interact according to narrative structures. While we are constituted through the range of stories available to us at any given cultural and historical moment (and the stories of the mentally ill have been particularly prescribed), narrative psychology, which emerged as a new paradigm in the 1980s (Bruner [1986] 2005; Polkinghorne, 1988; Sarbin, 1986), would maintain that we are also constituted and scripted through how we interpret, adopt and reject certain threads of these stories. But if this urge to 'story' is in some way hardwired, then this would suggest that we are also hardwired to tell some*body* that story, even if only an imagined body, as in some of the testimonies of psychiatric patients prohibited from having contact with either others or paper on which to write their stories (Hornstein, 2009). So we are back to a model of the human being as narrating and reflexive, and as inherently communication-seeking in both those quests.

This offers one clue as to why people want or need to tell stories and report some benefit gained in the telling. Through telling our story a sense of authorship may be felt, a temporary sense that we can re-script, *become* – and the sense of agency and possibility that accompanies this. As Ricoeur (in Wood, 1991) puts it, evoking Socrates, the 'examination' of a life occurs in its recounting. I don't live my life, examine it and tell it as separate enterprises. The living, the examining and the telling are concurrent, and happen δια one another, to use the Greek prefix, as in *dia*logue, meaning through; across; throughout – in a dynamic interexchange and interdependency.

Ricoeur (in Wood, 1991: 30) suggests that hearing a 'story not yet told' offers the possibility of producing a better story, 'more bearable and more intelligible'. In the eruptions of 'something else', where something beyond words and consciousness emerges and jolts the listener, but more crucially the teller, into a new way of thinking and even being – identity is evolved. Narrative also urges the speaker and listener to consider what does *not* get said, where emotions and experience fall outside words, and why the pause. Why the silence. Why the sigh of exasperation, as a last verbal resort, where words are not enough and the ineffability of experience overwhelms.

But there is more to narrative, especially when the narrative has been shot through with, or fragmented by, mental illness. This experience is described by Stone (2006: 44) as a 'radical disruption to a settled sense of identity, a felt impression that selfhood and being are under imminent threat of complete disaggregation'. Where there has been a history of trauma, as was the case with many of the people with whom I spoke, 'an experience of dissociation and disembodiment disrupts the traumatized person's sense of themselves' (Frie, 2011: 56). In such cases the narrator may have the experience of shattered or absent coherence. This experience is one far beyond that described as the lot of the postmodern subject, in which, nevertheless, as Crossley (2000: 528) maintains, 'a lived sense of coherence, unity and meaning normally prevails'.

Ricoeur (1986) describes narrative identity, in which the self only comes into being in the process of telling a life story, as taking place in the dialectic between order and disorder. In this space, or collision, the narrator, as Crossley continues, 'attempts to reconfigure a sense of order, meaningfulness and coherent identity'. This seeking of coherence, of a sense of going-on-being, despite the ravages of illness, the disassociation of trauma, and the imposition of the discourses of stigma, pathology and exclusion, demonstrates the resilience of the narrative imperative. It may offer a further clue as to why people with such disrupted trajectories were, and are, willing or compelled to tell their story. This quest for a coherent narrative identity also suggests to us a further means through which to understand the role of art practice.

Art and narrative identity

Any talk about people's voices should also recognize silence. That of the voices that did *not* speak to me – either out of reasoned choice, inability, unwillingness, or a possible sense of futility and despair. The silence of those who did not step forward to give their story or who thought about it but doubted or feared or suspected – those who, for good reason, did not want to be interviewed, prodded, extracted, re-presented, possibly exposed, criticized, analysed. They had been there, got the t-shirt. *No thank you.*

Let's say a word too about the silence of those with whom I began an interview that did not continue. There would be a short introductory stream of speech, invariably sounding rehearsed, tired; *well-trodden narrative* – which was then followed by a pause, a sigh, a shrug, a shake of the head, or other gesture of submission. Submission perhaps to a task that was felt destined to lead nowhere and would fall desperately short of what was wanting to be said – the 'genuine perplexity and frustration in the face of phenomena when trying to find the proper description for them' (Spiegelberg, 1982: 693). For these people, whose silences need to be 'heard' in this book, the pressure to abide by narrative coherence, linearity and order was experienced, perhaps, as inimical to the expression of their experiences of mental illness. Where do you start, really, to describe some of the depths and darknesses of mental distress? Where do you begin to pull together the fragments? For if narrative can offer a coherence, a sense of an identity on-going, it can also throw into relief the abyss between experience and worded description, or worse, the abyss between who I feel myself to be and the words I hear tumble out of my mouth. The story may have immediately sounded to the narrator as though being spoken through someone else's mouth, already a sedimented narrative. Perhaps it was felt to be steeped in the powerful discourse of the biomedical story, a story which occludes alternative identities, alternative understandings and wherein language tyrannizes precisely through it absorbing us, as Harper (2002) suggests, into these dominant ways of thinking. Then, in the interview space, there would come a withdrawal, an apology, and a story untold. As much as people can narrate their way into being, we are also silenced out of being, self-censorship, of all censorship, being the most dangerous kind. At the day's end, cultural forces determine what sorts of stories get told, basically, 'who gets a life' (Couser, 1997: 77).

Much of this is guesswork – I have only snippets of explanations from those who did not want to speak. But any presentation of what is said carries with it questions about what is not said, as any personal narrative is counterpoised by one not given. And in the withdrawals and untold stories is the *imprint* of many stories; of lives not listened to, of experiences, betrayals and hurts silenced; of language profuse in its inadequacy, of words slippery and duplicitous. For some, a lifetime of being mis-told, misrepresented, misinterpreted and re-scripted by professionals, carers and family members whose narrative is adjusted to make sense of their own task or pain, has led to a mistrust of language, especially its spoken form. The trouble with words, after all, said dramatist Dennis Potter, is you never know whose mouths they've been in. Or, one might add, whose ears they are going to land on. Psychology is rife with stories of people protesting their sanity and becoming labelled as lacking insight or being non-compliant. No shortage of stories, too, of the harsh penalties of what Rosenhan in 1973 described as the 'stickiness of psychodiagnostic labels' and how, once given one, every utterance in the psychiatric system is seen as further evidence of the diagnosis. My interviewees sometimes appeared over-careful and self-conscious in apologising for behaviours they worried might confirm, in my eyes, a defect, a disorder, an instability.

In the withdrawals, reluctances and untold stories is a key as to why art is turned to with such an unbending loyalty and gratitude. It doesn't require speech and language as such, and yet when it expresses what you want to say, or, more poignantly, what you had no intention or consciousness of wanting to say, it has the experience nailed more accurately and *to the bone*, than the richest of vocabulary. Words, on the other hand, are as Bakhtin (1981: 294) put it, always 'populated with the intentions of others'. The post-Kleinian analyst and theorist Wilfred Bion describes the sheer weight of emotion breaking up the words and expression of one of his patients:

The words that should have represented the meaning the man wanted to express were fragmented by the emotional forces to which he wished to give verbal expression; the verbal formulation could not 'contain' his emotions . . .

(1970: 94)

Over and again, people who did speak with me described the experience of symbolizing a felt emotion or experience in a way that words did not allow, or under which weight, words fragmented. As Liz put it:

So all the art work and all the healing that has happened in the last seven or eight years has really been about trying to find another language for the thing I didn't know how to talk about or the thing I didn't have language for . . .

Phil Baird, a 54-year-old artist, reflects on how experience can be carried in an image, and how that communication is timeless:

I grew up in Yorkshire and Scotland . . . I began drawing at an early age . . . I remember one drawing in particular which was of me picking snowdrops . . . it was about the **experience** *(pause) . . . I don't know . . . (pause) . . . well I found the drawing thirty or forty years later and it sort of . . . I could* **remember** *the* **experience** *of it . . .*

(emphasis in the speech indicated in bold type)

Phil's speech in this narrative is important to note; it is halting and intense. In speaking of the language of art, words appear to fail him, to fall short. Like very many of the interviewees, when speaking of art and its contribution to their survival or their *going on being*, there are many pauses, and pauses of varied textures. There are breaks to take time to choose a better-fitting word and exasperated paralinguistic features such as snorts and exhalations or ironic short laughter. There is the body, too, of course, rushing in where words end – with shrugs, creased faces, slumped shoulders and the fidgeting, mobile, making and unmaking hands. Often the narrator would become impatient with me, unsurprisingly, as though the subject at hand could not be described. Yet this point of Phil's, of an image expressing an experience better than words, is one that crops up the length and breadth of artists' stories. Such images were felt to express an experience in some way seminal. Seminal because it held an important part of one's autobiographic journey but also because in the process of making art, unknown or concealed experiences and their attendant emotions emerged and *then* became speakable. In becoming a part of one's storied self, these experiences and emotions became part of one's narrative identity which in turn 'made' something of these, in an iterative autobiographic journey – accessed, expressed, re-integrated – through an art practice. As Mabel described:

. . . worlds that exist within you can be revealed through the making and the painting and the drawing . . . it's something there that you've made, it's given you a connection with something outside of yourself but nevertheless part of yourself. That's the value of it.

Poonam, a 46-year-old British Asian woman, put it this way:

> *I believe in art – and I think it believes in me. It helps me access parts of me that don't have an opportunity to be expressed in my life. I feel I can be who I am when I create work . . . it includes the whole of me – and I don't compromise – in the way I do with the rest of my life. I trust myself when I make art. When my mum died I couldn't make any new work and felt frustrated by the awful attempts I made at drawings – but I learnt to accept that I just needed to pass through this barren time. In some ways it was useful to see that I was broken inside – something I couldn't express in words – and didn't seek out help to do this.*

Tara, a 47-year-old reclusive artist whose description of forty years of psychiatric interventions makes for hard hearing, says simply that the story of things that happen to us is '. . . *deep, too deep for language, but not too deep for the eye*'.

The idea of a picture speaking a thousand words is one we are all familiar with, but these narratives suggested even more than this. They suggested that accessing experiences, those remembered or those previously forgotten, as with childhood memories, and those previously inaccessible (some spoke of pre-verbal memories), was an essential part of their developing or restoring a sense of 'I'. In this developing identity, a reconciliation with oneself after, or through, a mental illness was being forged, and an autobiographical journey, not possible through other means, was being undertaken. This experience of *congruent* expression, felt to be a consonant part of one's narrative, seemed to cement a sense of identity, of I am. The making of art as well as the symbolization through imagery of lived experience, memories, and emotions afforded a sense of relief:

> *. . . my art helps me to connect to a part of me that was lost when I was very young. That part of me which was lost when my mum left. I was four years old and although I cannot say for certain I think I can actually remember the day that she walked out. Anyway I guess because I was then left with my very old father who was by then fifty-seven years old . . . this was by the way 1969 . . . he was very Victorian in his ways and views – children are to be seen and not heard. So as I grew up I had to find a way of escaping from this tyrant . . . I was never allowed to go anywhere unless it was with him and up until I was fifteen I was very afraid of my father . . . so the only thing that I found was art. So art has played a very big part in my life from a very early age. I think that experience really set down the foundations for me to become an artist. So now when I paint or create any kind of art I feel that I am talking to that little boy who just wanted some attention from his mum but could never get it . . . I believe I get in touch with a very sensitive very hurt part of myself and that through the very act of art I am telling myself that it will be okay and that . . . and not to worry. I feel that for most of my life I have been at war with myself, my art has become the place where I try to reconcile that war between the lost little four-year-old Paul and the grown-up Paul, the father and the mother.*

(Paul Ashton)

This relief and reconciliation is particularly poignant for many for whom there has been a disjuncture between the lived experience of illness and diagnosis; between one's life and the medical versions of one's history; between one's felt distress and the psychiatric language which describes it; between the human suffering and the medical discourse – just a few areas where what sociologists Passeron and Bourdieu (1990) called 'symbolic violence' was wrought. When this disjuncture, fleetingly or temporarily, receives reconciliation by the coalescing, at last, of experience and expression, it is powerful balm. Here is Ruth:

> *And I think that for me, that's where art . . . (pause) . . . you can actually explore your feelings through art much more openly actually, you can explore feelings of pain, you can explore wounds, you can explore how things are connected in a way that words don't give you the ability to or actually where words stop sometimes.*

A rationale behind the power of accessing our full store of memories comes from both psychoanalytic theory and narrative psychology – but it is also present in current research within the brain sciences, with a particular focus on the potency of accessing good memories. Previous research has suggested that being able to recall detailed memories that are positive or self-affirming can help to boost positive mood for people with a history of depression, and researchers are now looking into ways to help people with depression to recall happier memories with greater ease (see, for example, Dalgleish *et al.*, 2013). Whilst the narratives overwhelmingly described how art helped in the accessing and bringing to light of troubled and troubling memories, there were references to gaining '*a more whole picture*' (Yelena), and '*balancing the stuff I remember . . . it wasn't, no, it wasn't all bad . . .*' (Zot Dow). Indeed, in later stages of narrators' art practice, which I look at in the next chapter, this shift, through one's art practice, to a more compassionate view of one's past is sometimes identifiable.

But symbolic representation of one's experience appeared to be only one element of a package that was instrumental in the narrative identity role of art. As narrating beings, we seek to express experience, be it an early encounter with snowdrops or the harrowing depths of depression. This need to express emerged in the narratives combined with a desire to *externalize*. This externalizing element of art, found throughout the narratives, suggests a further component of one's narrative identity – that this is forged in relation to an other. Sasha, in the extract below, was by no means alone in describing the ways in which severe mental illness erodes communication and even a sense of being human. Having experienced this kind of bleakness, the expression and communication properties of an art practice were spoken of with effervescence:

> *You uncover . . . (pause) something in your experience and then put it together . . . and then you communicate it and the satisfaction is . . . phew! . . . em . . . sometimes when I'm communicating it I'm thinking God, what the hell am I going on about? I'm not understanding this, it's meaningless babble . . . but you come out the other side of that and then you get a connection with another person. My illness has come out of not being able to communicate . . . not even knowing what I could communicate, my illness was . . . (I say was, because I do put it in the past these days) was, completely inexplicable and inexpressible, so therefore if I can find a way of communicating with people and expressing things – much*

of what is connected to that illness is not being able to communicate . . . then it's hugely satisfying . . . 'cause it feels like something has come out of that horrible, wretched process – and it's about it's being human, I suppose, when I was ill I believed I wasn't human, that was a core belief . . . so that's why it's such a big deal for me . . .

In understanding this process of expressing one's experience and of accessing parts of one's history, externalizing these and entering into communication, it is useful to refer again to Ricoeur's concept of progressive and regressive hermeneutics. Ricoeur (1970) suggests that a dialectic is at play in artistic practice. A dialectic between an exploration of one's current and one's future life and that which is rooted in the past, which constitutes not 'just' an autobiographical project or an excavation amenable to the psychoanalytic space, but a project of going on being, of projecting one's self ahead. This identity-building process plays a vital role in understanding the passion expressed for the practice of art, almost independent of an enjoyment or sense of accomplishment obtained through the final product. This project of building a narrative identity is one which, in looking forward from the position of creating, holds within it potential – for change and for being other, but most importantly, for going on being. Stickley and colleagues in their 2007 study of mental health service users involved in arts activity similarly found that value was placed on the opportunity to develop an identity as an artist, and the hope that artistic expression gives participants.

Akerman and Ouellette (2012: 385), in writing about Ricoeur's progressive and regressive hermeneutics, suggest that 'artists serve as models for us all as they draw upon the past and transcend it both to lose and to reconstruct the self and identity'. This sense of forwardness and continuity was deemed vital especially after the lived experience in mental illness of disintegration, or even of annihilation. This sense of future, in the regressive and progressive movement, may provide one reason why in several of these narratives of art practice a dissatisfaction was expressed with talking therapies, compared with the autobiographic process often entered into through art making.

Talking therapies and speaking wellness

All the people with whom I spoke, with the exception of four or five, had had some experience of talking therapies, covering between them, predominantly, the modalities of psychoanalytic psychotherapy, psychodynamic counselling, humanistic counselling, Cognitive Behavioural Therapy (CBT), Mindfulness Cognitive Therapy (MCT) and Dialectical Behaviour Therapy (DBT). Some could not say what type of talking therapy they had had, either not recalling, or never having had it described and named to them. There was a caution in many of the narratives, in which interviewees who had had talking therapies said they did not want to appear negative about the process. Phil's exhortation that it was '*oh, way, way better than just getting more meds . . .*' was commonly shared, as was taking responsibility for *not* having found the process of talking with a therapist helpful. This was exemplified by Myra:

Look, he was a nice guy . . . I don't want to be negative. Maybe I just didn't get it. But I was at a point then . . . yeah, maybe that was it, I wasn't at a point where I could make use of the counselling, the therapy . . . and I felt stuck there . . .

Myra was one of several people who spoke of the experience, often the sensation, in therapy of being *stuck* – stuck in a story; at a point in time; stuck in a repeated micro examination of a particular problem. Kleinman (1988: 180), in writing of illness narratives, described the chronicity that he observed which 'arises in part by telling dead or static stories, situating the individual in a wasteland', while Roberts (2000: 438) remarks that the perpetuation of such a narrative 'exchanges the precarious and uncertain struggle for health with acceptance of meanings that forever constrain the individual's hope and potential'. It was just this experience of telling, retelling and perpetuating dead or static stories that was described by some as their experience of therapy. Here is Don:

Oh nice, yeah . . . we sat and talked, she asked me a few things, gave me time to answer and all that . . . listened . . . but I felt I wasn't kind of giving what 'was required' [makes scare marks with fingers]. I had told my story, loads of times . . . didn't really feel like going over it again . . . no, just didn't feel it was helping . . . didn't really know how to move it on . . .

There were also what appeared to be apologies, expressions of guilt, even, for not having 'tried harder'. Here is Kayleigh:

Um . . . I wasn't ready. And I had, you know, attitude . . . like, didn't want to engage. Saw her [the therapist] as yet another health professional, when really, I guess she was only trying to help . . . (pause) but I felt I had to kind of perform . . . something, to meet what was being asked of me, again, compliance, like another request that I behave . . . yeah (pause) maybe I should have given in a bit, as she wasn't like, a shrink or anything . . .

Ambivalence about the talking therapy route was expressed in a number of ways, and it was difficult for me to reconcile the person in front of me, explaining the limitations, the awkwardness, or even the perceived occasional harm of counselling from their viewpoint, with what I imagined were the words entered into their clinical notes when they had withdrawn from the therapy; words such as 'resistant'; phrases such as 'lacking in insight', 'refusal of engagement', lacking in 'Reflective Functioning', or even indeed, 'non-compliant'. Within a psycho-therapeutic paradigm, these may well be valid assessments, but the narratives of these 'resistant' people suggest that there was more to these non-fruitful therapy encounters than such notes might imply. Perhaps lurking behind this reluctance was a lack of what Peter Fonagy and colleagues (2007) have termed 'epistemic trust'. This trust, laid down in our early years and subsequent reciprocal trust-worthy interpersonal experiences, may be marred by the kinds of early childhood experiences most, if not all, of the interviewees shared. These experiences are compounded by mental distress, not to mention the jagged relationships such distress draws in its wake. The therapeutic relationship and its work may be undermined, according to Fonagy, by a lack of acknowledgement on the part of the therapist of the consequences of such an eroded or absent *basic* human trust.

These narratives also bring into question a commonly held belief that an analytic journey can only be undertaken through a professional intermediary. The rejection of therapies, rather, seemed to be one way in which individuals asserted themselves, resisting the language of psychotherapeutic discourse and its processes, and even words themselves. Sometimes this was out of sheer exhaustion with having told their story over and again to a raft of professionals. That did not mean, however, that there was a rejection of either analysis *per se*, or interpersonal relationship. But once an art routine, however small, however modest, had been established, it appeared to be offering a more consonant and 'owned' self-analytic process. In this, spoken words, with their trickery and inadequacies, played a smaller part, and at this point there was even less of a draw to talking therapies. Artist Connor, on reflecting on a history of mental illness and painting, reflected on the fact that:

> *If I had to choose what helped, in order of preference, I'd go for art practice, first, way over and above. Second, art therapy and last, way behind, but still on the scene, counselling . . .*

One way of understanding this choice outside of the psychoanalytic paradigm is in terms of the already mentioned dissatisfaction with the 'approximate' nature of words, and their potential to misrepresent, and be misinterpreted. This is particularly pertinent to people with whom I spoke, who, as part of early childhood experiences of sexual abuse, had not only developed difficulties establishing trust, but had also been caught in a web of lies, misinterpretations and silences about the abuse, sometimes stretching well into late adult life. While psychotherapy might indeed be a tool through which to provide a corrective emotional experience and nurture trust not only in another human being but in the very language with which such a relationship is built, some of the narratives of the way an art practice functioned suggested that this was what was felt to be provided by art; a means by which to build trust in an other and a language of expression and representation. And it was provided through the deliberate choice of the individual concerned, at a pace which felt comfortably regulated, and through processes and non-verbal media which offered the safety and staged exposure desired, as I will describe further in Chapter 6. Most of the narratives did indeed describe a self-analytic process, one which was also risky, even frightening at times. But this process was felt to be occurring in a space created by the artist and owned by them, a process that allowed a vital sense of stepping outside the medical discourse, outside the therapeutic paradigm in which they were to be 'treated' as patient, client – *the ill*. This, going back to Ricoeur's concept of progressive and regressive hermeneutics, was fundamental to the building of identity. Art provided a bridge between the 'old' identity, with its trauma, its illness, its diagnoses, treatments and medications, disavowals and 'chaos narrative' (Frank, 1995), through the self as survivor, someone 'in recovery', towards being something else, something more. For some, like Leonne, who declared themselves an 'artist', the very word held all of these stations of the journey: '*Being an artist, having arrived here . . . **there's** a creative project! (laughs).*' Others felt they 'weren't quite there yet', and although they were still hesitant in calling themselves artists, they did know they had become something other than victim, patient, client, *ill*. As Connor put it, '*through finding a way to paint it, I had become something more than*'.

This newly forged identity helps us to understand why by far the most prominent 'complaint' about the experience of talking therapies was, as Crystal said, that they kept you '*talking about the same stuff, and completely going round in circles*'. Ruth too, in recalling her experience of counselling, alluded to the belief that we create ourselves through what we speak of. She felt very strongly that a positive framing of 'the problem' was important for her, as was a sense of beyond. She had felt pressured in the therapeutic domain to produce a narrative, a vocabulary and expression, of 'problem':

> *You are looking at the problem, all the time. All the time, it's the problem. The illness, the symptoms, the trauma . . . I needed to step out of that, to look away, no, to look ahead . . . I needed to speak well-ness . . .*

This nod in the direction of the relationship between our wellbeing and our narrative emerged frequently in participants' narratives and is an important theme in both narrative study and positive psychology. The study of possible correlations between how we speak about our lives and how we feel about our lives is ongoing (see, for example, Bauer *et al.*, 2008) and inconclusive – but we should be cautious of a quickness, within our therapized cultures, to accuse those who do not wish to ruminate on the past and its distress of being in denial or in some way lacking the fibre to confront their demons.

With their lightened allegiances to exploring the past, cognitive behavioural approaches were found by a few to be 'helpful' – in the short term. Tilly described CBT as '*a management programme, really, helpful, but I can't say it gave me any deep insight . . .*'. So there is a difficulty here, yet again, a falling short; on the one hand insight and exploration were spoken of as desirable, but on the other, a repeated excavation of the past was deemed unhelpful. A sense of weariness is felt again, with words, the 'client' role and the clinical domain – and the narratives resound with a struggle; a grappling for some other way, means, language, process, by which to explore, analyse and confront. A few saw CBT as 'didactic' and as setting them up for yet more finger wagging, of which they were tired. There was an anxiety expressed, too, by a few, about the '*little tricks of failure*' if they didn't approach the various 'tasks' properly. One person caustically likened this to going to see the hygienist knowing you'll be asked if you have flossed, and knowing that yet again you haven't: '*Yep, one more failure . . .*'

Talking therapies were in no sense rejected wholesale; and useful points were raised about how the experience might have been made more fruitful. In some of art making's intensely private moments, to which I will return in the following two chapters, the accessing and expressing of pain, for example, was described. Painter

Phil Fry says that art *'lets me bleed off excess emotions'*. This sheds light on why, for a few, talking therapies had begun to make more sense *after* they had begun exploring the extreme end of painful and traumatic experiences through their art, in an arena in which they could control the exposure and the disclosure to some degree and become more fluent with the material of the pain. Some claimed this process allowed for a language to emerge that they could then more productively use in therapy. Gladding and Newsome (2003), for example, have noted the use of arts as a means to facilitate counselling, and there are further implications for the use of 'art *in* therapy' as distinct from art *as* therapy (Edwards, 2004).

This reintroduction into the 'linguistic community', with a return to language heralding a 'cure' from the 'desymbolization and denarrativization' of illness (Ricoeur, 2012), is commonly thought to be the realm of analysis, taking place within the analytic space. But for those who had formerly rejected either the process of talking therapy with its high premium on words, or its relational aspect in which they felt enmeshed in yet another relationship experienced as asymmetrical, or its perceived discourse of deficit, pathology and illness, it is significant that one of the uses for art practice which was 'stumbled upon' was this: to express, externalize and process some of the rawness of lived experience, and prepare one for engagement in therapy. Marty, who suffered severe and repeated abuse as a child and a youngster, described it thus:

> . . . a lot of my past history of therapy . . . (pause) I really hadn't been ready, I wasn't in a place to talk about it. I wouldn't say it was a waste of time but you have to be ready and you have to find the right therapist . . . And because my mental health was informed by being abused as a child, it's just taken me lots of years to be able to bear to talk about it. And I can do it now, but only because I've used my art as a vehicle for expressing it . . . in my last therapy sessions I took my drawings . . . so what I could . . . uh . . . verbalize, was there on paper to be picked up on.

Sarah is an artist in her twenties, now training to be an art therapist. She has suffered both a history of mental illness and surgery to help with severe epilepsy. She described what began as an unhelpful therapeutic alliance:

> . . . talking therapies can sometimes dance around a subject . . . we were completely, like, **missing** each other . . . and so I started to get frustrated with him and I found the sessions pointless . . . I found it really frustrating . . . em, I just . . . found it . . . I couldn't find my words . . . (pause) . . . I'd have this feeling that I kept losing my words . . . I'd have the therapist sitting in front of me kind of looking at me . . . and he'd ask something like 'how are you feeling' and I **knew** but I just couldn't say and I found it was really pointless . . . but we got past that . . .

(emphasis in the speech indicated in bold type)

Sarah invited the therapist to her exhibition, and to her evident surprise:

> He came! Which I think was a real turning point in our relationship . . . my respect for him grew enormously, em, and I think also, he, I don't know if it helped him . . . see my work, but that was like a turning point and after that I was able to use the sessions better . . .

Another artist, Harli Tree, who has been diagnosed with Dissociative Identity Disorder (DID), spoke of the dynamic, bi-directional work of talking therapies in tandem with her art practice. Here, the psychotherapist was '*talking to the other personalities*' while the very young personalities, who do not yet speak, painted their experience. She found this a crucial part of enabling her to live with her DID and was hopeful for this process continuing – but insisted that it was the art that enabled this progress:

> *To start with they [the personalities] never used to do anything together, now the main 'alter' has communicated with the rest of them and sometimes they do the art together. Which is good because it means we're coming together as one. Hopefully, I won't need to split off into different parts, and hopefully I can become one person, one personality . . . not going to get rid of them as such, but we can all . . . it's hard to explain . . . this might have been achievable to somebody else by other means, but for me, it's more achievable by producing the art . . .*

All of the people with whom I spoke described feeling that they didn't '*work well*' in words. And while this was not borne out by the often highly articulate accounts people gave of their life and work, as well as occasional references to writing poetry, perhaps one of the most important messages in the narratives describing experiences of talking therapies is that the very material of these therapies, the spoken word, is to some at best second to the materials of creating and image. The philosopher Susan Langer (1895–1985), who continues to inspire psychoanalysts, artists and art therapists, spoke of art as articulating the very shape of human feeling in a way words can never do, arguing that language is an inadequate means of capturing the essential features of conscious experience. She describes how, for example, in a painting, 'the balance of values, line and color and light . . . is so highly adjusted that no verbal proposition could hope to embody its pattern' (Langer, 1930: 160). Language, Langer maintained, 'is almost useless for conveying knowledge about the precise character of the affective life' (1957: 91). That it is a means particularly weak at describing the affective experiences in mental illness is a view expressed repeatedly in my interviews with artists.

The arts therapies clearly have a hugely important role to play in mental wellbeing, but once again, their activation through the clinical, therapeutic, and even 'social and collaborative' discourses serves, it would seem, to alienate some people for whom art *making* is part of their identity. For them, the art practice has to be wrestled away from these domains, as I described in the previous chapter. It has to be slowly chiselled into something theirs, something which operates symbiotically with a developing narrative artistic identity.

Recovery and discovery

One of the reasons people were willing to tell me their story was that they had reached a point where they felt well enough and defiant enough to put that story on the table. Some of the silences and the gaps where stories could have been were those of people who were very unwell, or had relapsed into an episode of mental ill health which had pulled them back into a voicelessness, a period seemingly known to each narrator. During such a period, in Jil's words, you just had to '*stay put, stay quiet . . . batten down the hatches and try and survive . . .*'. Certainly people felt there was a role for medication, even hospitalization, and that sometimes the depths of despair were plumbed and you emerged again by using your own resilience, gritted-teeth determination, or whatever other strategies you had. So it is beholden on anyone interested in mental wellbeing to explore the many ways used by people to get out of that dark place and to the point (again) of being well enough to 'tell it'. One of the ways that emerges in the narratives I gathered is through an articulated or implied belief in the tenets of the recovery movement.

It is worth considering the impact of this belief on people's lives, looking at its meeting point with an art practice and identifying traces of recovery discourse in the narratives. This discourse was detectable in people's stories and appeared to enable an alternative life narrative to that felt to be 'expected' of someone with a history and diagnosis of mental illness. In itself, the recovery discourse offered a narrative of resistance to the labels felt to have been applied before – schizo-phrenic; patient; service user; depressive; or any one of the abundant and often deprecatory labels which circulate so forcefully in society.

The narratives gathered in this research fall largely into the category that psychologist Dan McAdams and colleagues would term 'redemption' narratives. In these, 'the storyteller depicts a transformation from a bad, affectively negative life scene to a subsequent good, affectively positive life scene' (2001: 474). As such, they were formulated through a move, linguistically, to frame the negative into a 'positive' – as mentioned earlier on in this chapter. The narratives also can be seen to fall into the third of Arthur Frank's (1995) categories in his classification of narratives, the 'quest' narrative, in which a journey through suffering is described, one in which adversity is now being faced head on, in the belief that something is gained, or to be gained, from the experience. Both types of narrative are saturated with recovery imagery, terminology and symbolism.

One of the emerging themes from the narratives is the idea, consistent with this approach and nutshelled by Ruth who we met earlier, of 'speaking wellness'. It went hand in hand with an emphasis throughout the data on looking forward, and, as has been described, an emphasis on being or becoming *other* than the illness. In today's therapeutic culture wherein we increasingly construct our problems in professional, medico-scientific language there is concurrently a more positive, agentic discourse of 'recovery' and autonomy in operation. This is shaped in part through the accounts of people with the lived experience of mental illness, people like Patricia E. Deegan, psychologist, researcher and activist, once diagnosed schizophrenic, who have become known as 'experts by experience'. Such first person narratives and a process of storying one's journey are central to the recovery paradigm and have played a significant role in both forming 'recovery' and informing it. It is now widely endorsed that policy and mental health services embed a recovery orientation, and in England mental health policy has explicitly supported a recovery focus since 2001 (Perkins and Slade, 2012).

Not surprisingly, the literature on recovery and the penetration of its concepts is vast.[2] There is no one definition of recovery, but a wide range of definitions, some grounded in a medical model, others in a more grassroots approach. Bill Anthony is the author of the most widely cited definition of recovery as:

> a deeply personal, unique process of changing one's attitudes, values, feelings, goals, skills and/or roles. It is a way of living a satisfying, hopeful, and contributing life even within the limitations caused by illness. Recovery involves the development of new meaning and purpose in one's life as one grows beyond the catastrophic effects of mental illness.
>
> (1993: 15)

A cluster of broadly aligned principles have motivated, reassured, inspired and galvanized huge numbers of people with mental illness. Particularly widespread in the UK, Canada, Australia, New Zealand and America, the recovery movement offers a counter-narrative to the psychiatric and medical 'story' of mental illness, one which 'belongs to consumers-survivors, not to practitioners' (Schiff, 2004: 212); it is a forceful narrative, and shares with positive psychology a belief in the power of looking ahead and in scripting a new identity. It is based on principles of acceptance and resilience, on strategies for living and on hope and empowerment. These messages of a fundamental strength and tenacity in the human being certainly resonated for me, having spent the past few years talking to mental health 'survivors'. And this book is one more testament to the self-strategies developed or encountered by people who have reframed their lives.

By approaching the narrative data thematically, themes common in recovery discourse can easily be identified: 'acceptance' (of one's illness and one's history); 'identity'; 'belief in recovery'; 'hope'; and 'strategies and management of illness'. These themes mirror some of those found in the review of the British literature on recovery (Bonney and Stickley, 2008) and are those which are easily, perhaps, co-constructed through individuals' exposure within a given culture to recovery literature, its practices (even as performed by mental health professionals), peer groups, and the many and varied community groupings and projects described in Chapter 3. It is nevertheless important to try to see what use was made of this discourse in conjunction with an art practice, and whether an oppositional identity was enabled. How did this narrative of recovery appear to intersect with that of an art practice? And how did the practice itself embellish or redefine the narrative?

Now, one's narrative can be life-affirming, and we can energize a sense of self, rescript an identity, focus on ahead and a stronger way of life. But it can also hold and reproduce toxic stories; indeed people alluded to this when they spoke of the limitations of therapy, and being wary and weary of fossilizing illness-dominated identities (Scheff, 1999). They believed, in some cases, that such stories would condemn them further – echoing cognitive-based self-help strategies and positive psychology, edicts of which emphasize proactivity in the course of redefining one's future as somewhat freed from the shackles of the past. It should be recalled, however, that earlier extracts in this chapter are taken from a wide selection of descriptions which also speak of connecting through art practice with the past and one's hidden 'demons'. The progressive and regressive autobiographic process of Ricoeur holds that this movement forward and back, collecting, remembering and meaning making, is part and parcel of narrative balancing. But art, it seems, in its making and at times unmaking, through its destruction or rejection, offered a conduit for this connecting and 'handling' of one's fragments from the past, and I will describe this further in the following chapter. Amidst the many references to recovery made by artists was a strand of narrative that described, or tried to describe in often inchoate and halting phrases, how art practice and recovery were interlinked. As Neenah put it, '*My art practice has been very central to my recovery – it has been there, in tandem.*' Tamsin spoke of recovery from different bouts of illness, rather than as an ongoing 'programme':

> . . . *when I was in hospital, one of the ways I slowly recovered, myself, I'm never sure how much medication helped, was to go out and start painting again, so after I'd done those very raw and painful therapeutic paintings, I just went out and painted every day just the surroundings around the hospital and that's what enabled me slowly to get well again and to forget myself.*

Yelena was cautious in over-attributing wellness to the role of art, but was clear that for her there was a connection:

> *Does it help my mental health? (pause) . . . it's a difficult question because mental health, to answer you honestly, mental health to me is so confusing . . . It is absolutely impossible to encompass it and I can see the limitations of art; I can see the limitations of anything compared to my mental health because when I see the art I can see an image but I can't see the whole picture. It never is the whole picture. Does that make sense? So it doesn't give me completion and I don't think art will give me completion. It won't create an answer. It won't give me recovery. (pause) It **won't** give me recovery. It is not a cure . . . is what I'm trying to say. But it is a process and during that process I see myself getting better . . . so I guess it does, [help] . . . yes.*

For Solange, making art ensured that she 'looked after herself', another important tenet of recovery. She had to make sure she was 'well enough' to pursue her passion, which, by the time we spoke, was also her profession:

> *It does help recovery because you try to be good with yourself and accept yourself with everything. You feel you're you at your work, you grow your confidence and identity, you're showing who I am in a way. You're being open with yourself, and that helps.*

Here Darrell questions the idea of 'recovery', but then also endorses one of its principles – acceptance of who you are and what has happened to you:

> *Personally I don't know about recovery. I find the whole concept of recovery dubious. I'm not sure you can recover from certain things. I think the things that have been key in my life, the*

issues that have been plaguing me throughout my life – I don't think you can therapize those things away. I think you have to just kind of live with them. They're part of what makes you what you are.

Marty and Ruth echoed other participants, who, when speaking of recovery, linked it to the being with others. This was a being involved with the *recovery* of others, and this involvement took place through their art and the types of community projects described in Chapter 3:

. . . art and creativity in general are definitely part of my recovery so I do my best to use it to help other people empower themselves. I can't explain how it works, it's not quantifiable, and you can't work it out from statistics and attendance records. It's a bit mysterious.

(Marty)

So KindArts was set up by myself and other people who also had mental health issues who also used their art work to help them recover.

(Ruth)

But Ruth later added a caveat about how and where people 'recover', alluding to the social determinants of health:

But yeh, . . . well they know that people in poorer communities suffer higher levels of ill health than people in richer communities and also will recover differently . . .

People also referred to their 'recovery journey' and its meanders. They described an acceptance of their illness and of what had happened to them, which in some cases was harrowing. They spoke of insights into this journey gained, in some cases, exclusively through the making of art.

But to what extent was the 'recovery' discourse yet another potentially limiting, or even toxic, narrative? And did an art practice do anything to undermine this? In their critique of the discourses of recovery and resilience, Harper and Speed (2012) bring to our attention at least three salient points regarding the infiltration of discourses of recovery. First, they argue that the concepts of recovery and resilience are individualistic, based on medicalized and neo-liberal notions of individual responsibility. Secondly, Harper and Speed suggest that resilience discourse continues to be implicitly reliant on a model of deficit. The recovery discourse, they argue, 'simply reframes deficits as strengths and is thus implicitly reliant on deficit-based models' (Harper and Speed, 2012: 10). Finally, they note that structural inequalities are routinely de-emphasized within the neo-liberal framework. In terms of a macro analysis of how discourse works in our lives, positioning us to take up an identity and a voice through these discourses, this is critique we need to heed. Its sober message reminds us to ask, always, whose interests are served through the propagation of any given discourse.

The emphasis on the individual in recovery can indeed be seen as part of the neo-liberal package, hand in hand with the Big Society, with its crafted versions of community and volunteerism custom-made to enable a shrinking welfare presence. This is the shrinking welfare in whose retreat the inequities of health and wealth are worsening, and there is indeed a vested interest in having people who may be ill believe themselves well. In many of the narratives I heard, this sense of individualism was compounded by the enduring notion of artist as individual, as I have mentioned in the previous two chapters. Yet this lone-artist allusion was almost always countered by descriptions of the interpersonal nature of one's art practice; you communicated to somebody; an audience's response was highly valued; art practice needed you to 'get out there' and get connected, apply for grants, enter competitions, team up, show up and hang up. So while the 'I' in the narratives of art was paramount, that 'I' seemed to become a 'we' as one's art practice progressed – sometimes to the surprise and even elation of the interviewee, as the following chapter will describe. Here is Paul Ashton on the importance of the communicative role of his work:

> *Ultimately I want my art to say something. I don't want it to be a little pretty cottage picture on a wall somewhere. I want people to interact with my art. I want people to see it and feel something about it. Emotionally being moved in some way. Even saying, 'that's a pile of shit. I could do that.' That, to me, is a response. That's what I want. I want people to look at my art and feel moved by it, and to walk away from the gallery or wherever they might have seen it and think to themselves, that made me think about such and such.*

But did an art practice in any way unseat the 'deficit' contained, nevertheless, in the recovery discourse? Returning to the silences implicit in the 'voiced' of this research, I wondered how many of the non-story-tellers were burdened or 'erased' by pressures of the recovery discourse. What happens if, for example, you are not feeling empowered? If you feel that your story does not contain evangelical proclamations of resilience? That in fact you *are* ill; and stuck in a bleak space where you cannot communicate, reach out, share, 'manage' your symptoms, or even get out of bed – all of which has been richly described in accounts of the depths of illness, rather than its recovery. Then how do you begin to position yourself in front of a veritable army of survivors, policy makers, and professionals all chanting Recovery and Resilience? How much more of a 'deficit' is your illness now that there is, apparently, a step programme of recovery, and you just are not on it? So it is important, in any narrative work, to 'hear' the silent voices, and be mindful that one woman's positive narrative may well place another woman's in *deficit*.

Many of those with whom I did speak had no illusion about the recurrence of mental illness. Some seemed acutely aware that they shift from one side of this narrative divide to the other, swiftly. They referred to the inconstancy of health and, as art maker Poonam put it, how '*I can say this now because I feel well . . . can talk to you now . . . that's not a given for next week, or year . . . even for tomorrow.*' Recovery, in any of its definitions and manifestations, is precarious. And, as with other forms of severe illness, when in remission, the body and mind seem to do what they can to erase the memory of pain. There is a tendency also to 'idolize' one's recovery strategies, even one's art practice, and denigrate non-art interventions, therapy included, a tendency that can also be identified in some of the more zealous narratives.

Yet for some, particularly the 'veterans' of art practice who could look back on more than a decade of committed art making, there was indication of the art 'bringing things together', of 'integrating' and helping the artist usher in a more nuanced view of her history, his battles, their illness. I will return to this in the following chapters to take a more psychoanalytically informed view of the mechanisms through which this 'quest for integration' may be taking place.

So the narratives gathered for this book speak an overarching 'language' of recovery. But such language, when funnelled into an art practice which provided a reflective, rebellious, sometimes confrontational space, appears to have been efficient and instrumental in helping some individuals move away from the pernicious psychiatric discourse of terminal pathology still based on a Kraepelinian pessimism. It also seemed to facilitate an engagement with the political – once again through the processes of self-analysis and expression that appeared to be the foundation stones of people's art practice. The interpersonal in art practice, at whatever level this was spoken of or alluded to – be it a conversation with one's abuser, an imagined spectator, through an arts community, potential buyer or indeed a therapist – served as a catalyst for positive social transformation.

> *I know now, what I felt then [in the psychiatric ward] but only because I've drawn it, looked at it, drawn it, looked at it, and finally felt it. And only now, can I say 'that did that to me – that system, that way of dealing with illness, did THAT to me' . . . it was a revelation, and I couldn't step back from it. I couldn't now do nothing . . .*

> (Keith)

To unpack this a little further, let's go back to a point made earlier, that art practice enabled both an expressing of experience and emotions, and an accessing of these, previously not remembered, or disavowed, perhaps. Although what I want to illustrate is not by any means confined to one person's narrative, I want to take the example of Mink, whom we met in Chapter 3. Diagnosed with DID in 1994 and first hospitalized at the age of 14, Mink spoke about her thirteen *painting* personalities and how each engaged in an art practice unique to them. Mink has been involved in art for many years, and has a substantial practice, with a body of work, exhibitions and collaborations and media coverage as part of it. In a fascinating interview where Mink speaks of her experience of DID and the painting of thirteen different personalities, which, as she laughs, puts the idea of collaborative art in a whole new light, she alights briefly on one who paints with bright colours:

> *I learn a lot about the others [personalities] . . . she [one of the personalities] paints with bright colours and she says . . . it's because with child abuse, people ignore it . . . and take no notice, and yet with the bright colours you can't miss it . . . I wouldn't have known . . . about the abuse . . . she apparently had been told not to talk about it . . . well, she's not*

talking about it, she doesn't talk, but she paints it . . . I've come to understand them better . . . but it also made me feel closer to them . . . because I felt this is part of them on this canvas . . . because I'm never going to meet them . . . because we're not co-conscious . . . so I'm never going to really know these people but I did feel closer to them . . . especially when I had the first exhibition, and I stood in the gallery looking round at all the different styles and the different personalities' work on the wall and I thought this is the closest I'm ever going to get to them.

For Mink, art is a 'part of who we are' and it is a practice which is not only part of her (their) autobiography, but one which *is* the autobiography. But the practice continually challenged her, bringing more material to the fore, demanding that names be named, blame apportioned, actors in the complicated story of who they were be identified, symptoms considered, and both the personal and political strands of their narrative addressed. In such a profoundly complex disorder as DID, it is hard to imagine another means by which these personalities could be accessed, and through which they each would explore, to a greater or lesser extent, the conditions and circumstances which led them to silence or to dissociation.

Another artist, Katie, also described how images and thoughts emerged as she was painting 'something quite unrelated', which led to her reassessing her psychiatric history and the role of her family and others in it:

I kept coming back to being in hospital – over and again these images would present themselves and I just started wondering . . . how did I get there? What was I doing there, nineteen years old, without anyone asking me, really talking about what had happened? That all seemed so wrong, suddenly, but god knows why it took so long for me to ask that . . .

What is important to note in these, and many of the other narratives, is that art practice is not 'easy'. It is not a leisure activity (though it certainly has elements of relaxation) and it is not 'fun', although narratives were not devoid of either the humour or pleasure sometimes experienced in art practice. What did emerge, time and again, in the narratives, were examples of self-reflection, self-analysis and confrontation, through the art making. Connor, a mid-life painter, claimed that as in meditation, regardless of what you meditate *on*, what comes to the surface *is your life.*

Whilst I am engaged in making art, I also spend a lot of time thinking about my life, the direction I am taking, relationships, regrets, etc. It's all there . . . laid bare . . .

This was spoken of as involving risk, in the self-reflection and in the disclosure; and demanding honesty. Sometimes these reflections led to direct and painful acknowledgements of the forces arrayed in opposition to mental health; the discrimination, inequality, poverty – and the increasingly bleak impacts of unbridled market forces which simply demanded that many of us stay ill. It led, in some cases, directly to action, and to harnessing one's experience to that of others, in short, to a politicization of the story. As put plainly by Ayden, '*They need us to buy their drugs . . . buy into their therapies . . . we being ill makes them well . . . I started seeing that . . .'*

One theme running throughout the narratives seemed to give the artists in this story particular trouble in verbalizing. This was precisely how their art practice was 'autobiographical' and how the dialogue between the art and one's wellbeing or one's illness was articulated. On the one level, there were direct descriptions of how at an earlier stage of their art practice, *'everything was just stuck up there'*, which was Leonne's way of describing the *'purge 'n' tell'* element. This gradually gave way, in most cases, to a slower, less 'explicit' symbolization, to which I will come back in the following chapter. But what was unequivocally described was a belief that not only was their work autobiographic, even when it did not explicitly deal with motifs from their own life, but that it *was* their autobiographical journey – *'I am my art practice'* was heard often, or, conversely, *'my art practice is who I am'* – which certainly echoes the way narrative is said to function: we are the stories we tell and those stories feed back instantaneously into who we are (now) and the practices that are us.

Artist Andrew Locke, diagnosed as schizophrenic and currently involved in the movement to re-classify and rename schizophrenia, presented the art and autobiography 'package' in this distinctive way:

I think . . . (pause) I think I actually got ill to make art, I think it was a conscious decision as a nine-year-old boy that I wanted to make art and there was something simultaneous about illness that happened at the same time and that's been the duality of what my art making has been for me. This balance between this absolute passionate desire to create art that simultaneously makes me unwell, or maybe not unwell, perhaps unhappy . . .

It is interesting that it is my artistic discourse that is enabling my wellbeing, and let's hope, a continuation of my recovery. This idea I mentioned of a flight from oneself to create, so that a sense of togetherness with myself would help me feel whole again. My whole experience of this illness could be seen in that way. Insight is precious, as is remaining creative, and I am interested in the connection here . . .

Phil B, a painter who has been diagnosed with schizoaffective disorder, put it this way:

I think my art and my mental health have ended up being so intertwined it's really hard to tell them apart . . . I think probably for a long time, em, I thought they were separate things but of course they're not 'cause the work is always about the state of mind that I've been in . . . so, I don't think any artist makes anything other than autobiographical work, no matter what it is . . . whether it's Rothko's big pictures, or Picasso's paintings, Monet, Manet . . . Warhol . . . sighs . . . (pause) (laughs) I mean if Damien Hirst's Shark isn't a self-portrait I don't know what is . . . (laughs) but for a long time I didn't think like that, you know I thought art was your one thing and then you was your something else . . . does that make sense?

And Stevie, a young art student with a history of severe mental illness and multiple bereavements, appeared to struggle hard to put this into words, reminding me again of the approximation of all these stories:

> *it keeps me on the ground . . . it um, keeps my feet on the floor and it keeps my head level . . . and it . . . it helps me . . . you know be who I am so . . . you know I had really to sit back and think how I was going to do it and I could have continued the whole course drawing flowers, butterflies . . . you know creating a past that was I don't know . . . you know . . . what was socially acceptable . . . um but that didn't help me ultimately in my life . . . Art has been there as my body . . . Art has been my . . . Art is my whole entity. I am who I am because of art. So . . . and . . . that's what all my painting is about . . . it's about doing and . . . not getting . . . not becoming ill . . . it's to deal with the situation . . .*

It seemed that the recovery narrative took people so far; but it was the art practice, initially fortified by recovery principles, which then took these people beyond the rhetoric, enabling a narrative of connection. It was also a narrative of greater resistance, insight and power which in many cases had led to direct activist involvement of one sort or another; resistance and insight because of the self-analytic journey which appeared inevitable through a sustained art practice (even for those who had shunned or eschewed this element to begin with); and power because two things appeared to be happening. First, a more coherent narrative identity was apparently forged, and second, this vitalized, integrated self was experimenting with interpersonal manoeuvre and in many cases functioning more efficaciously within wider social relations. In the next chapter, I look at the nuts and bolts of artistic activity, digging more into how the process of making art contributes to the autobiographic project and wellbeing.

Notes

1   There is a lively and provocative debate within qualitative research regarding the extent to which psychoanalytic concepts such as transference and countertransference can be actively used as research tools. Readers are referred to Parker (2010) for a critique, and to Holmes (2014) for a useful review and extension of the main points of the debate.

2   Readers are referred to *The International Review of Psychiatry*, special issue, 24(1) (2012) on 'Recovery around the Globe': http://informahealthcare.com/toc/irp/24/1 (accessed July 2014); and, for an important critical overview, Harper and Speed (2012).

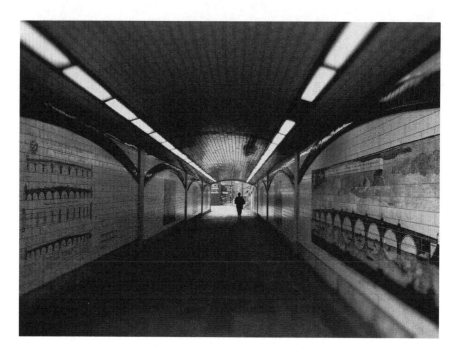

Tunnel vision

5   Art making, unmaking and repair

A new result is of value, if at all, when in unifying elements long known but hitherto separate and seeming strangers one to another, it suddenly introduces order where apparently disorder reigned.

(Henri Poincaré, 1910)

The people whose narrative extracts appear in this book were at very different points in their recovery or discovery journey. Part of that journey, as described in Chapter 3, involved pulling their art practice, sometimes haltingly, out of the clinical setting, away from the confines of 'mental health art' or even the discourse of 'community art'. Participants spoke fervently of not wanting to be categorized, pigeon-holed, or consigned to any one label, and of being driven to self-determine. As Charlie Devus put it, '. . .to become an artist allowed me to live on the peripheries of myself – to reinvent, perpetually . . .'.

I wondered whether perhaps it was this same defiant, independent trait which had helped these people emerge from the bleak childhood experiences often described, which gave them the resilience to get to the other end of the dehumanizing psychiatric corridor and the strength to carry on the journey. Part of this journey, too, as I described in the previous chapter, was a discovery, recovery or initiation of an artistic narrative identity. In this journey with its multifarious battles, art making played, and was still playing, a central role. And while participants were insistent in describing what they were doing as 'not art therapy', making art was always spoken of as being therapeutic. Whilst this semantic hiccup may well indicate that deliberate positions had been taken up outside formal therapeutic and clinical processes, also revealed is the affirmation that making art very often simply makes people feel better.

Because stories were unequivocal in this affirmative support of art as therapeutic, I wanted to pursue with these people how art was *experienced* as therapeutic. What did this mean? How was this benefit experienced in temporal terms? Here the conversation would often be busy with pauses, shrugs, silences, head shaking and hands raised in open stance expressing the ineffability of the experience. Yet beyond the many phrases like '*I can't really explain it . . .; it's hard to say, exactly . . .*', which suggested that such an experience is 'better felt than telt', a cluster of experiences did nevertheless emerge in the descriptions. Overall, these experiences chime with current research which suggests that art making is experienced as beneficial in relation to the cognitive, in relation to the social and in relation to the affective dimensions of mental wellbeing, and that through these art participation contributes to overall resilience and wellbeing (Royal College of Psychiatrists, 2010; Stacey and Stickley, 2010; Self and Randall, 2013). These benefits and their domains cannot easily be disentangled; the temporal, spatial experience of making art affords minutely varying benefits in different domains at different times, and this repeated contact with the experience accumulates over time to produce transformation (DeNora, 2013). In this chapter, however, in order to look more closely at the experiences described and their constituent elements, I will separate the benefits into different domains in accordance with how, in the narratives, people described the 'felt' impact. I will begin by looking briefly at descriptions of benefits which may be loosely regarded as 'cognitive' – drawing these from where participants described the impact of their practice, broadly, on their thinking.

One of a range of such thinking benefits that were experienced and described involved the 'derailing' of negative thinking patterns (Camic, 2008) and the 'distraction' process involved in this (Drake and Winner, 2012; Secker *et al.*, 2007; Parr, 2006). Here is Sue talking about how her work:

> . . . *keeps my mind off my problems . . . it's relaxing . . . intricate patterns give me a way of stimulating my brain to think . . . there are a lot of problems that can't be sorted out right now . . . but I can process my thoughts this way, it gives me time to think, and I actually find I can remember more things because I relax . . . when I'm doing art I'm not thinking about anything else, my problems, or housing or welfare or my next appointment with social services . . . it's just me and whatever it is I'm working on . . .*

And for Pauline:

> *Art acts as a distraction. Unless I am really depressed and empty, as I have found myself recently, I find that when I am engaged in my work, viewing exhibitions or simply talking about art I am not struggling with negative thoughts . . . I become absorbed.*

Yelena also appreciated the way art derailed her mind from its 'buzzing':

> *Well, it quietens the mind. It creates positivity and it brings forth positivity and it makes me feel positive and excitement. How does it do that? I don't know. Well the concentration part is the part that quietens the mind; can you understand that? It is not like my head is buzzing when I am painting. It is the opposite.*

Lauren, a young woman recently diagnosed with a personality disorder follow-ing a suicide attempt, described some of the difficulties she had already encoun-tered by the age of 24:

> *I had been suffering from depression all through my teenage years and although I was doing everything I could to feel better, medication, counselling sessions and CBT courses, nothing shifted it and I knew there was something else wrong with me.*

For her, art making enables a trance-like state which previously had been experienced when in violent, charged situations such as physical fighting:

> . . . *It's therapeutic for me, when I really get lost into something I am doing, and this sometimes feels like I am in an almost meditative state. This leaves me feeling relaxed and I think it helps with my spinning thoughts as I can focus my mind on just one thing and not worry so much for a bit. I find it helpful to have a safe place to comfortably 'let go'. It's really hard to explain, it's . . . erm . . . I'm not thinking, I haven't got any kind of . . . intrusive thoughts going on, it's quite peaceful . . . and, it's usually if I'm doing something quite detailed that I get into that kind of trance state, something quite repetitive, it's really relaxing and I feel I can just let myself go a little bit . . . (pause) it's a similar feeling to when I used to get into fights, it's that kind of trance state, but with painting, it takes the edge off, stops the panic and anxiety . . .*

Lauren was not alone in describing an intertwined cognitive and affective experience. Many participants spoke of an experience which had the characteristics of 'flow' as described by positive psychologist Mihaly Csikszentmihalyi (Csikszentmihalyi and Csikszentmihalyi, 1988). In this state, the activity itself is intrinsically rewarding and there is a merging of action and awareness. But Parr (2012: 7) cautions us that when talking about creative experiences in a mental health context words relating to trance-like states may be 'misread as symptomatic of mental instability'. This again reminds us of the ways in which language can be hijacked, and how experiences that are 'acceptable' in a given population (non-mentally ill artists) may nevertheless be regarded with caution if not suspicion when described by those with histories of mental illness, a sad reflection, perhaps, of our inability to hear and our quickness to pathologize. Taking people's descriptions at face-value and exercising no such clinical or suspicious censorship, it seems that artists' narratives described a range of experiences which were life-enhancing, unique and seemed to advance their connection with their art. But there was also a reticence, at times, to enter into more florid descriptions of what to some, like folktale artist Adena, were *'quite simply states of grace . . . given to me, gifted to me, while painting . . . but I can't really say that to my psychiatrist . . .'.*

Felix, an Eritrean painter, describes his experience thus:

> *To stop the brain . . . in that way it helps me. I could be in a room . . . anywhere . . . when I am painting what I am doing is all-encompassing, I am all drawn into it, and I am not trying to dictate what I draw. I want it out. It is beyond restriction. It's like spiritual things. This is endless.*

Such 'flow' states are typified by a focused texture of engagement and are characterized by feelings of contented absorption where there is a suspension of thought. Here is Chloe Shalini:

> *The best time is when I've started a piece and have got into the 'flow' . . . am working intuitively, less consciously.*

> *. . . it is receiving or feeling an intuition that is . . . it is so large it feels almost as if it is coming from outside of you. You know it's not but you almost feel as if it is and I get a sense of like a light above my, not exactly above my head but sort of . . . but only very vaguely – in a very kind of inner vision sort of way and [it's] very much a feeling of certain elation, but a very calm feeling at the same time, nothing manic or anything. The way that you feel when you just know that something is right and you get a kind of calm, or security almost.*

There is an ensuing loss of a sense of self and of time, and participants who referred to distraction sometimes elaborated on this point by referring to a 'slipping into' a 'meditative' state:

> *. . . it is when you are completely immersed in the moment . . . afterwards it's like coming out of a long meditation and you can feel so overjoyed . . . and it also gives me confidence and aspirations . . .*

> (Yelena)

For some, this experience had spiritual resonances, with descriptions of 'merging' with something bigger than one's self, echoes of what Freud (1927) called the 'Oceanic'. He traced this feeling back to an early phase of 'limitless narcissism' from which he determined we should progress rather than regress. Yet returning, however fleetingly, to the core of the infant's experience of unbounded merger with the mother and with the world – neither of them formulated yet as separate entities – may well be experienced as pleasurable relief. A well-known principle, after all, of many recovery and self-help programmes is an acknowledgement of something 'bigger' than us, with which to connect, through which to let go and by which to take a new perspective on the demands and persecutions of ego. Such a sense of 'flight', pleasure and release may well return us to a pre-verbal expansiveness and offer an explanation and theoretical psychic mechanism through which to better understand Csikszentmihalyi's 'flow'.

Description of this 'merging' experience in art, lived through with such intensity perhaps because it re-conjures pre-verbal experiences of oneness, is terrain well-trodden by psychoanalytic theorists. Ellen Spitz, Professor of Visual Art, suggests the art encounter:

> . . . may temporarily obliterate our sense of inner and outer separateness by drawing us into an orbit in which boundaries between the self and the other, and also categories into which we divide the world, dissolve.

> (1989: 142)

This distraction, 'flow' and apparent removal of consciousness from the present, conscious and embodied state provided a sense of release and relief for many who spoke with me, describing a move into a place where the *'thinking stops'*. In some cases this move 'elsewhere' was spoken of more concretely, in relation, for example, to the mundane drudgery of a locked ward. Here, as Yelena put it:

. . . painting is a way of finding something interesting to do and it kind of gives you a sense of who you are again and a sense of beauty in this kind of terrible, terrible situation. I think it was a way of trying to find something that wasn't so ugly around so that I had something to focus on . . . when I was in hospital doing art I felt the benefit then because it was relaxing. It was meditative and it was a way of getting outside of my mind. So the process was relaxing and the process was meditative. It took a lot of time. Time was so slow in hospital. Time seemed to tick by. Five seconds was torture but while doing a painting it took up an hour and I was like, 'Wow, an hour has gone, fantastic. An hour less in hospital.' So in that way it was an occupation that was good for the soul and relaxing as well as taking time up that was a really difficult situation.

In such settings, it was all too easy for, as Leonne put it, '*your mind to start going to bad places*', and in such instances art making offered a reliable place in which the mind could rest, maintain its own focus, and even, in 'flow', take flight:

Well, being in an ex-lunatic asylum in a semi-secure unit is very frustrating and the days are long. Whilst I'm in my art my day floats by . . . it's rewarding as well . . . (long pause, sob) I start with just looking at an image and I think I can reproduce that in pencil, or in pen . . . people see my feathers that I draw and say they feel they could pick up, they're so soft . . . when I work, I smile . . . I feel joy, a radiance of heat coming through my body. It's like the sun coming up . . . it's a warm, glowing, rich feeling going through my body, does that make any sense? It's such a relief, of stress and er . . . any aggression or frustration or anger that's in me . . . I get to sit down in a quiet place and just relax and draw, it's incredibly therapeutic.

(Gerald)

The private, and carefully guarded, domain of art making, especially when occurring within secure units and hospitals, was almost revered as providing a space where, as Ella said, '*your mind is free . . . protected from what's going on . . . art helps me to get back to me*'. Parr (2006: 156) similarly found references by the artists in her study to an 'interior creative space' that functions as a 'safe location that can be accessed as part of a strategy for recovery'.

The artists in this study who spoke of art practice in this way seemed not to be dedicated to any one particular type of visual art making or medium, as though it was the process, the experience and the relished private space they entered into when making art that offered them respite. Here is Paul Ashton:

I'll draw, paint, make pots whatever they give me to use, I'll use . . . I'll draw a bird one day or a beer can, doesn't matter . . .

There were other cognitive benefits also spoken of in relation to having this private activity and space. These included having '*more orderly thoughts*' after such an experience of art making, being calmer in one's speech, or enjoying sharpened concentration, and for Ella this was '*despite the damage done to that through the medication*'. Any one of these experiences may also have led to the attendant physical benefits sometimes described (Teall, *et al.*, 2006) as a result of the relaxation and calming effect reported. On occasion, however, art also impassioned, even enraged, dredging up the forgotten or disavowed past in its wake and throwing up its debris all over again – a point I will return to later on in the chapter.[1]

On the whole, these narratives again lend weight to conventional understanding of how 'art works' – helping the mind and its functions, even if it is on the relatively basic level of '*getting my mind off stuff. . .*'. For some, art as distraction from troubling environments, mundane routines, bleak thoughts or painful memories provided an effect experienced as therapeutic, and they were content to stay with using art in this way, allowing them, as for Vita, to '*bury myself happily in what I love doing*'.

For others, this private domain of art practice with its distracting and calming qualities changed over time. Some people with whom I spoke felt, on reflection, that they had needed the distraction less as gradually other areas of their life gained strength or other occupations took hold and wellbeing and self-understanding were felt to improve. So art as distraction offered a time out from troubling thoughts or periods of drudgery and listlessness and was one way in which people felt better. It cleared and calmed and relaxed, through routine, through its patterns, composition or colour. But for many artists, there was more to the experience of making art than getting a mental time out. Some described art making as performing an ordering and integrating role, and I want now to turn to this strand of the narratives and explore it further.

Ordering and controlling: sifting the 'I am'

As described in the previous chapter, a sense of order and feeling of control were highly valued by most participants. This is perhaps less than surprising given the numerous ways in which mental illness was felt to have wrecked order and splintered any sense of an ongoing identity, echoed in accounts in the literature of mental illness more widely. Stone (2004: 18), for example, suggests that such illness is characterised by 'fragmentation, amorphousness, entropy, chaos, silence, senselessness'. From such frightening places, art was often seen as offering a means by which some control could be reasserted and some order perceived.

Here is Jayne, in her words, '*an obsessive drawer*':

> It [art] just helps . . . I felt that when I was at my worst I felt that I didn't have a voice and I wasn't able . . . (pause) . . . I was able to say things through my art work that I wasn't verbally able to say. It just empowered me as a child as well as an adult now. I could tell people things that . . . (pause) . . . I was silenced as a child . . . but I could still draw. So I still, I could still, I still had some control in, it just, it just gave me some power and even now today I still find it really therapeutic to just be able to express myself, if I can't do it verbally I can always do it through my drawing.

Illness and trauma were thus often spoken of as having led to a deep sense of being out of control, first of one's mind, and then, once within the confines of a regime of diagnosis, medication, monitoring, perhaps sectioning – of one's body and life. A welcomed sense of order was described as a feature of both the process of art production and the product itself, offering a direct impact on how one felt. It was this more immediate experience of order that was spoken of as being instantaneously beneficial, rather than therapeutic over the long term. For some, including Jasmine, a young painter with a history of mental illness and a past of deeply troubling life events including psychotic episodes, night terrors, and frightening hypnagogic imagery wherein she lost all track of what was 'real' and what was not, feeling out of control was a watermark of her childhood and young adulthood. For her, even hospital routine was welcome, because here:

> *I felt safe. I knew when to wake up, I knew when meal time was, it was the sense of routine that kept me safe, I was in control again . . .*

She now speaks with contagious relish and effervescence about her many art projects. Yet in contrast with their zany and exuberant nature, this sense of order and safety remains paramount:

> *Art has always been a refuge, something I feel safe doing . . . it gives me a sense of purpose, order. It's something that makes me happy to be me.*

For Liz Atkin, a long-term compulsive skin-picking condition meant that control of the medium, her environment and what she chose to expose or display of her condition, her body and her art was an important element of the work:

> *. . . so my compulsive skin picking, which has been in my experience for a long, long time in sporadic episodes, has existed for more than twenty years . . . and I understand it to have come very much from those early experiences in the home when I felt very out of control and the only thing that I could control, I guess, was my own body and my own encounter.*

> *. . . I often work with the camera in my hand, it's an immediate transaction, photographing transformed sections of skin. I work with all kinds of different materials to create new textures on the body. This process is creative rather than damaging . . . light is a very big thing in photography, and I am illuminating the body. With control over the light and use of the camera it's that sense of control which remains . . . is quite important in the work as well – that I control what is seen by the audience once the work is finished.*

For some participants this sense of order was sought and gained through the concrete *routines and rituals* of art, as well as in the 'order' of the medium. Here is Pippa Lee, an avid colourist:

> *. . . the fact that I have this area, a physical space in my flat, where all my lovely art things are . . . it's one space that feels truly me. But I also feel . . . I dunno, relaxed, I think, as soon as I start mixing the paints, even the touch of the brush . . . and I tend to approach the work using the same routines, which soothe me, immediately . . . Of course it [the paint] doesn't always do what I want, but oh the joy of getting it closer to the order, the way I want it to be . . . can't describe it, when that paint goes on right, when the colour is just spot on,*

when the texture is as I want it. How do I feel? Calm, a sense of order, not just with me,
with the universe! (laughs)

The completion of the art piece, sometimes through to its '*point where it just tells*
me it's done', as Pippa Lee continued, or to the point of hanging it on display, was
described as playing a part in the sense of order. Seeing your work '*become part of*
the cultural scene', as Phil Baird put it, and thus part of a larger order, outside yourself,
was described with surprise, wonder and pride. But such finality was also described
as offering a further point in the sequence, a '*tidier order*', as Adena suggested, '*a loose*
end of me, my story, not solved (pause) but seen, held, tied . . .'.

This welcomed sense of order experienced through making art was also
described as stemming from transforming inner chaos into an outer ordered and
tangible form:

> *. . . I had no way of expressing what was going on inside. Home life grew worse and I felt*
> *inner chaos, the flashbacks and panic attacks were destroying my ability to function, to be*
> *able to live at all and I was so ill with the bulimia, in various ways. Painting in this way*
> *enabled me to extract a more manageable portion of the chaos outside of my head so I could*
> *look at it and somehow digest and transmute something terrible into something that, although*
> *not necessarily aesthetic, something of value, a 'good' from a 'bad'. At least it gave more*
> *lasting relief than self-harm.*

(Chloe Shalini)

The interviews presented a picture of individuals engaged in a struggle against
this sense of a fractured, disordered 'I' – against what Kristeva (1989: 33) vividly
called the 'excess of an unorderable cognitive chaos'. They were full of descriptions
of the ways in which art was instrumental in offering a sense of clearing, order and
control. Here is Ruth:

> *. . . one of the pieces of work I did, when I was living in Germany . . . I collected hundreds*
> *and hundreds of plastic carrier bags and I then washed them and hung them up on a washing*
> *line. And I kept doing this kind of washing of carrier bags and I still think that's a really*
> *important piece of work that I did, for me. And probably most people think well that's quite*
> *a strange thing why would anyone collect carrier bags and then wash them? But I actually*
> *think that's quite important in terms of our sustainability that we actually keep these carrier*
> *bags and we do wash them. But also carrier bags are also about what's going on in here,*
> *(points to her head) there are carrier bags of detritus that we carry around with us all our life*
> *and sometimes we need to clean them out.*

As I described in the previous chapter, one of the ways in which it appeared that
art played a role in helping to restore a sense of order was through the formulation
of an ongoing narrative identity. This, you will recall, involved for Ricoeur a 'to
and fro' process of building an autobiography, with the work of art embodying 'a
disappearance of the archaic object as fantasy and its reappearance as a cultural
object' (Ricoeur, 1970: 314). Ricoeur suggests that in this dialectic, between

unconscious and past 'objects' and their reappearance as work of art, a cultural object, a narrative identity which draws on one's past but reformulates it into a present and future, is built. Ricoeur presented this in contrast to a classic psycho-analytic process which was largely a regressive means of understanding an individual. But today, in the light of post-Freudian object relations theory, an idea of progressive and regressive identity building can be understood in terms of rejecting parts of one's self, disavowing elements of one's history but then gradually re-introjecting parts which are nevertheless valuable to one's identity and a richer, more consonant sense of 'I am'.

This process seemed an inherent part of producing work which contained elements of one's history that had been forgotten, previously inaccessible or disavowed, thus allowing a renewed sense of the past and one's possible positioning in a future. It was integral also to the production and completion of the work itself and the reinvention of oneself as an artist, a 'new' identity which was experienced as empowering and congruent, as described in Chapters 3 and 4. In many cases this process of ordering and integrating was further reinforced by the narrative interviews themselves. This was the case particularly where the artist spoke to me more than once, over a period of time, and engaged deeply in the opportunity to reflect on their autobiographic journey, its linkages with their art, and to consider the road travelled. Here is Yelena, in the interview, looking back on the work she produced in hospital, and reconfiguring now how she feels about herself *then:*

> *So the work that I did there was the work that I remember the most because that was where I struggled the most. That was the hardest work I put into something because my muscles weren't moving; my mind wasn't working and so when I look at those pieces of work I really have a heart for them. I really have compassion for myself.*

This ordering, searching and sifting, which the process of making art enabled, was implicit in so many of people's stories. Whether it is part of the experience of mental illness to become a seeker and whether the seeking predates the illness or even exacerbates it, we don't know. But the range of experiences I heard described seemed to tell a story of people involved in a quest – for sense, for order, and for understanding.

In some narratives, descriptions of order, either of one's thoughts, one's inner world as it became transformed into a coherent image, or the calm felt after turbulent emotions were put to temporary rest, moved on to speak of subtle processes of *integration*. I want to look at these now, to try to get to the experience of what was being described.

Integration: saying I am

In much of the material describing the art-making process there were perceptible stages that were passed through. These began with the throwing out of a felt experience of 'mess', evoking what the psychoanalyst Elliott Jacques described as 'rapid-fire creative production' (1965: 229), and moved on to working with the transformed material, manipulating it into a deeper expression which was felt as a more profound order, an integration. Anton Ehrenzweig, in his classic *The Hidden Order of Art* (1971), conceptualized three phases of art production, a conceptualization which is still of use to an understanding of these episodes, and for what might be happening for the artist, internally, in each. His formulation has strong resonances with Kleinian topography that this and the following chapter make use of, so we need to gain familiarity with some of Melanie Klein's sometimes contentious words and terminology.

The first of these phases for Ehrenzweig (1971: 123) is that of 'schizoid fragmentation' in which material is ejected, spat out, as it were, in a fierce 'attack', in an attempt to rid oneself of 'stuff'; the thoughts, images, representations, experiences and fragmented parts of the self. Zot Dow called work done in this period his *'full-of-pain-pictures'*, and Phil Fry described how at such a time:

> *The way in which I apply paint to canvas can be very physical. I have been known to puncture the canvas on many occasions. I love the canvas and the paint, but I hate it in equal measure.*

And Tamsin, speaking fast and expressing this momentum with her animated hands, described how:

> *I had to get it OUT of me . . . it was good to get it out . . . I needed to say it – there – that's me: look . . . saying YES! I was ill, and the pain and nastiness of it all, was like throwing it back at the world for once and I didn't care or take care of what I was painting or how it looked, or whether it was 'good' or not . . .*

This externalization sometimes led to a period of reflection, suggestive of Ehrenzweig's second phase of unconscious integration. Here, previously unconscious forms are integrated into consciously perceived shapes, forms, images. Some of the artists I spoke with described the sometimes uncanny realization of what a particular mark, image, symbol or work had 'been about':

> *I'd recognize something in all that . . . it would be looking back at me and I'd be like, 'THAT'S what that's about' . . .*

> (Leonne)

For some, a period of less than conscious doodling or mark-making offered a segue, one that Pajaczkowska (2007: 36), drawing on Milner (1950), describes as enabling a release for the mind 'from conscious intentionality', in so doing rendering it 'receptive to other, less conscious states of experience'. Here is Jayne:

> *Doodling, yeah . . . it's as though in that doodling phase, stuff comes out, material, maybe images, a line, a symbol, form . . . maybe I didn't even know was there, and I'm looking at it, and thinking . . . hmmm . . . **I know you**. That then might get pulled into a drawing, a more formal representation, I guess you can call it.*

In her 1958 essay 'On the development of mental functioning' Melanie Klein describes how important it is that destructive impulses and unwanted, split-off parts of the self that give rise to anxiety and pain are gradually integrated. These parts are valuable aspects of the personality without which we will always feel depleted and without which our creativity is stymied: 'Though the rejected aspects of the self and of internalized objects contribute to instability, they are also at the source of inspiration in artistic productions' (Klein, 1958: 245).

As described in Chapter 4, participants described how *expression* was crucial as processes or forms, shapes, compositions, textures or images reflected back to the artist '*parts of myself*'. In this way art helped to access and to depict experiences from a life; those remembered, those previously forgotten, those previously inaccessible, perhaps even pre-verbal – and those which only came to light through the art. Here Martha Orback describes the way in which art will 'show' what is on, or indeed in, one's mind, externalizing material that is avoided or dreaded:

> *It was completely unintentional . . . em, and actually had been happening before I was kind of really conscious about it, I guess was searching for an explanation or a way of understanding some of the things that had happened to me . . . one of the pieces I made when I was still at art school, was about nightmares and the time when my mother's brother committed suicide, but I didn't really know that, when I started making it, I em . . . I just thought I was making a project about having nightmares when I was little . . . but you know, once you start working on it and also when you look back on it you kind of realize oh yes, that was the explanation for that. Another project was indirectly about suicide, but I didn't think about it particularly in those sorts of terms . . . but then when I, I was doing some printmaking . . . I started making images, and some of these images, with mono-printing . . . you keep overlaying and so . . . I was quite enjoying the process and I didn't start off making this image, about essentially what became an image about accepting the possibility of having to go on without people . . . that got . . . that turned up, kind of through this mono-printing session of overlaying and when I made it, I was like . . . I thought 'Oh – that's what I'm thinking of at the moment' . . . em, and, it just kept happening like that, I'd be working on something and I'd start somewhere else and end up at this point . . . because . . . someone in my family had just tried to kill themselves and that was in my mind, and that was what I was thinking about at the time, but it wasn't really conscious, it was just what was there at the time . . .*

Such bringing to the fore was felt to help integrate and bring to life previously disavowed parts of the self. This process of integration is not only forged in the making of an image, but in the making – and sometimes in the destroying and the remaking – process. For Jennifer, a quietly spoken, reserved young woman, a history of serious self-harm and cutting which left her scarred for life was addressed in her art making. In her process, she used suture thread to embroider her work, literally 'stitching together' delicate images which were then juxtaposed with other media to remind the viewer this was not 'just embroidery'. Here both the physical process of making and the image, which holds the sewn-up whole, addressed Jennifer's 'frayed' history; a body torn, and the need to repair:

It's [the art practice] gone more towards embroidery this year . . . it started off at the end of the second year, I was looking at more personal issues. I was looking at eating disorders and self-harm. I started doing a bit of embroidery with suture thread and that led on to found embroidery from charity shops and unpicking old embroidery. There was one piece I did. It was like an old 1950s embroidery of two birds. I unpicked one of the birds and sewed it onto a white blank canvas. I guess there's been a clinical aspect to it as well in that I was kind of looking at the clinical and the homely and the overlap between the two, and I think that was drawing on my experiences quite a bit . . . I didn't sit down one day and think, 'I want to make this about me' . . . I think there is definitely a stronger element of me in there than I would like to admit sometimes.

. . . I brought [you] some images of it . . . that was the embroidery bit, the bird . . . and that one was taken out of the space and it was . . . sewn on the white. It was kind of like the homely and the clinical, and the displacement, and the relationship between the two.

And Crystal, in the extract below, was not alone in describing how art delivers the artist to a point of choice – of parts of one's self:

I made another piece with clay which were two balls, one was pure curves and no pattern, completely abstract and the second one was a sort of sputnik or satellite, a circle with lots of barbs coming out, and that also reflected two different sides of my personality . . . the parts which were not connected. And through making more and more work that looked at the different elements, I was able to start to not only bring them closer together but start to see what was the me that I wanted to keep and what was the me that I wanted to let go of.

But sometimes the expression was of unwanted, unexpected images, memories or experiences. These, as Zot Dow said, would be continually *'reminding me of stuff . . . bringing me down, down . . .'*, and this was often experienced as destabilizing, even frightening. Yet if the artist can 'stay with' and tolerate this destabilization then sometimes a breakthrough can be made.

. . . at times what is experienced and expressed is not very pleasant . . . it is all part of the main working through [of] sometimes difficult experiences . . . it can be a good way of integrating and coming to terms with some quite difficult experiences.

(Phil Baird)

An appreciation of, and capacity for, staying with the unease and allowing a period of gestation is shared in both therapeutic and creative endeavour. It is through such an episode, as the psychoanalyst Wilfred Bion (1970) put it, that the unthinkable may become thinkable. He invoked the term of the poet Keats, 'negative capability', which is the ability to be with 'uncertainties, mysteries, doubts, without any irritable reaching after fact and reason' (Keats, cited in Bion, 1970: 125). This capacity for 'being with' uncertainty, with doubt, and with pain, is often thought of as necessary for both mental wellbeing and creative work. It is in the *inability* to manage conflicts and ambivalence that, for psychoanalyst and art theorist Hanna Segal (1974) amongst others, the roots of inhibitions in artistic expression lie. Artist, art critic and former analysand of Melanie Klein, Adrian Stokes, also maintained:

> But he [*sic*] cannot be an artist unless at one time he reckoned painfully with the conflicting emotions that underlie his transformations of material, the aggression, the power, the control, as well as the belief in his own goodness and reparative aim.
>
> (Stokes, 1965: 25)

And more recently, Maria Walsh described the role of art, again through a Kleinian perspective, in helping us work through a necessarily repeated anxiety and to tolerate it:

> This toleration can be broached through art practice where the artist is continuously producing and reproducing images and things that do not simply allay this anxiety but heighten it. But this heightening of anxiety in art is a 'pleasurable unpleasure'.
>
> (2013: 114)

Some individuals spoke of this sense of an iterative process in which they would take work to a point then retreat from it – digesting, perhaps, the onslaught of disruption it seemed to cause, but then returning to it and facing down whatever it was that stared baldly back at them. Sometimes this was a destroyed piece of work. Kayleigh, an artist who had a history of abuse and illness, described how:

> [*I'd work at it*] *over and over . . . it kind of . . . took hold of me. It wasn't pretty, the image, nor the feeling, but it kept recurring and I kept dealing with it and it kept defeating me . . . and I'd bin it. Only to come back to it. Eventually some sort of . . . er . . . penny dropped . . . about what I was trying to get 'right' [gesticulates scare marks] . . . it was about the body, my body . . .*

The ways in which we compulsively remember and repeat were first observed by Freud in his famous 1914 essay 'Remembering, repeating and working-through (further recommendations on the technique of psycho-analysis II)'. He claimed that repressed memories lead to a compulsive acting out of these, and this repeated acting can be understood as a way of remembering, a human attempt to relegate the 'incident' to a proper past, a *history* rather than a past in the present. Some of the narrative threads referred to what seemed to be such a felt compulsion and the experience of a repetitive quality in the art activity. Charly, a young painter diagnosed with BPD, spoke of *self-sabotage:*

> *If it's not through drugs and drink like before, suicide attempts, it's now through my work . . . like, I won't finish it, I'll wreck it, by doing something, either by just bad painting or by actually smashing it up, spilling something on it, whatever . . . and I'd never bleedin' realized*

before that that's what I was up to . . . all along . . . self-sabotage . . . don't complete, don't enjoy, don't achieve . . .

And here, Charlie Devus alludes to the flip side of repeating, in the service of art:

It's something I can't stop doing, I must do . . . (pause) otherwise I feel very, very panicky . . . it's very difficult to say what happens . . . to reinvent . . . the pathological will to create, well, it's opposite is the pathological will to destroy . . .

Psychoanalyst W.R.D. Fairbairn also explored art in terms of destruction and repair, and preoccupation with both echoed in many of people's narratives about how they 'treat' their art. They also sometimes referred to how their art treated *them*; creating, demolishing and remaking their identity, their self-esteem, self-belief, and their health. Fairbairn claimed that the destructive urges which he believed lay at the basis of psychic tension found relief through the production of art. Here is Ruth, echoing this:

The thing I think that's really important is you can be really destructive with art and you can be really angry with things. So for me that's a really positive thing. You know, like you have a lovely white piece of paper and you can destroy it and fill it up with something else and I think for me that's quite a magical moment that you can actually destroy something but come up with something that has another life. So it's not destruction that becomes just negative destruction whereas I think being unwell sometimes can become very negative and very self-destructive . . . I think this can be a destruction that then leads on to a positive end . . . there was one time when I was really extremely unwell . . . I couldn't concentrate at all, I'd lost my ability to really think, I was having real problems holding conversations. I'd got to the stage where I couldn't really hold any food down. I just wasn't well at all. And I managed to start tearing up paper, a bit like kind of just doing this action of tearing up paper and then I got to the stage where I was tearing up coloured paper and putting different coloured paper in different bags. So I collected all this torn-up coloured paper and I got to the state where I could actually then turn the coloured paper into pictures. And that's when I started getting well, was from tearing the paper and then being able to put . . . putting it into something and I think it was that ability to reconnect, to get my brain to reconnect into actually doing something. Because it's quite hard to explain and it's probably quite hard for most people to know that at times I haven't been able to leave my house, I haven't been able to hold a conversation, I might not have been able to sleep for longer than twenty minutes at a time, 'cause when you're really unwell it can happen you might sort of doze for twenty minutes but then you wake up again in a kind of blur and that does really destroy a lot of your cognitive ability and also your ability to do anything else really. But actually then being able to be very destructive by destroying all this stuff but then making it into something . . .

And for Liz too, there was a compulsive activity to the art work which brought elements of her illness into stark relief for her, aiding her understanding of her illness and also pushing the work itself on:

I ended up compulsively making this artwork . . . in the middle of the night which was when the skin picking used to happen and actually the practice began to align itself with the illness in that way and slowly it's something that has helped me recover and create work.

Yet this is tricky business – and a fine line to tread when the interplay between one's art and one's health, and between one's past and one's present, is so poignant. This pleasurable unpleasure needs to be held bearable, and not tip over onto the side of destabilizing one entirely. For while art can show us that we are not masters and mistresses of our own house and that the re-presenting of our past continues throughout a lifetime, the uninvited re-emergence of this past in our praxis can be tough to face. This aliveness of pasts of trauma, illness, neglect and pain demonstrates the courage involved in the making of art, a process, sometimes, of 'deep mining into the darkness' (Gabora and Holmes, 2010: 285). For some, the process of making art moved far beyond a distraction, beyond a means by which to express oneself, and into a quest for a more authentic way of living through knowing one's history, and one's present – better. Yet, as art historian Michael Ann Holly points out, a life examined always:

> . . . entails the recognition that hindsight hurts as much as it heals. Tragedies unforeseen, things that were not said, stories without conclusions, all lurk there behind us, forever insisting on more attention sometimes than our minds and hearts can bear.
>
> (Holly, 2013: xiii)

If such unease can be worked with and worked through, the artist may find movement, through the work, into the third phase of Ehrenzweig's formulation, that of 'depressive introjection' (again, the terminology is Kleinian), where 'the work of art assumes independent existence and "otherness"' (Ehrenzweig, 1971: 119). For Ehrenzweig and many other psychoanalytic thinkers, the artist's relationship with her or his artwork replicates features of the therapeutic relationship, with success in the three-stage process being indicative of health. The eventual acceptance of the work of art as 'other' is an achievement: 'If satisfactory human relationships are proof of mental health, as is universally accepted, then the creative mind is healthy through establishing at least one good object relationship' (Ehrenzweig, 1971: 108).

The making of art thus also produces a space between the artist and an 'other' (the group, the spectator) with a third thing being created. This 'thing' expresses a distinctive personal aesthetic, having passed through the self in relation and co-creation with an 'other'. Lynn Froggett, Professor of Psychosocial Welfare, has conceptualized this as the 'intersubjective third' or the 'aesthetic third' (Froggett *et al.*, 2011). This is an object dependent on an *exchange* – an idea we will return to in Chapter 6. This capacity for 'thirdness' is also the basis for reflective functioning, in which one is able to be in mediation with the social world, and in acknowledgement that an other exists with a mental state not identical to one's own. Widely considered an important ingredient in moving forward with mental wellbeing, this capacity is instrumental in managing the challenges of the Kleinian depressive position. The 'object' of the art production can also be thought of in terms of the transitional object (Winnicott, 1971), evoking the first not-me possession that originally substituted the primary caregiver. The negotiation of this developmental hurdle, the transferring of affection, identification and trust to an other, is thought to enable a symbolic association, one considered to be a cornerstone of an ability for play and creativity. A picture emerges of space and fluidity as necessary components of mental wellbeing and creative ability – a space in which one moves, symbolically, from an encapsulated 'me-ness' to an admission of the other, her/his imagined emotional world and the possible connections between us – forged through, in this case, an art object.

What is important here, and chimes so readily with people's stories and accounts of their art practice, is that these phases seem to present what is fundamentally a process of ordering and integration, a working through of object relating. They indicate how deeply linked our mental state is with the art process and vice versa, as 'stuff' is ejected, then taken back into ourselves, detoxified, to be re-introjected and integrated into the 'I am'. Here is Martha Orback:

> *It's a way of taking something which I experienced as deeply traumatic, horrific and messy and going . . . 'OK let's try and make something out of this', and the process of taking all that mess and emotional chaos through the kind of creative process of forming it into something which you're then happy to show, and can explain to somebody else, is quite profound . . . because those experiences of chaos and trauma are quite hard to explain, and so, em, yeah, I often found myself not being to explain what was going on, but through doing something creatively, er, it was much easier because I could talk about something, or I'd made it into a form that (a) I was happy to talk about and (b) I understood better, so I had more grasp of it . . .*

Descriptions of each of these stages emerged in the narratives, and appear as part of a process which is cyclical, rather than linear. As mental health exists on a continuum, along which we slide in either direction, so art was spoken of as capturing these positions, functioning differently at different times. But in order to 'trust' the art in this process, it had to be felt to be able to *contain* parts of the artist which were being ejected; in Ehrenzweig's (1971: 185) words, the work of art 'acts as a containing "womb" which receives fragmented projections of the artist's self'.

Containment, another word from the psychoanalytic canon originally from the work of Bion, is one which has long been employed within art therapy (Edwards, 2004). As an experience, this sense of containment was reported to be intensely beneficial, and warrants more thought here. For Bion (1962b) the feeling of falling apart and of sensing one's self in bits was fundamental to the human condition, a 'nameless dread', out of which, however painfully, emerged thought and creativity. In detailing working with psychotic processes in art therapy, Katherine Killick poignantly describes the falling apart and coming together of the deeply troubled state:

Faith, in the continuity of being which persists through catastrophe, allows those experiences of interplay between falling apart and coming together, tearing apart in order to build anew, which are essential to creative mental activity of all kinds.

(1995: 108)

Across the span of the narratives, people spoke to me of the experiences of disintegration and dread that mental illness rendered acute. These were characterized by sensations of disruption, chaos and void. Across these interviews there emerged and re-emerged testimony that art and its practice were felt to help integrate 'parts' and 'bits' of oneself:

I was falling apart . . . like there were, er, bits of me all over the place, didn't feel I was 'together' you know . . . when they say 'pull yourself together' (laughs) they've got a point, and art helps me do that, pull these bits together . . .

(Leonne)

The term 'containing' (Bion, 1962a) has entered popular discourse and is applied in many, sometimes confusing, ways. Nevertheless it is a useful placeholder to describe something which is felt to 'hold' us emotionally. For Bion, the infant needs the mature, functioning mind of another (ideally the caregiver) to help it tolerate and organize what can be overwhelming, if not frightening experience. Held by the receptive mind of the other, the overwhelming stimuli can pass through the 'container' and be re-delivered to the infant, detoxified. Consider the many instances when a caregiver will hear the cries of an infant, feel and interpret the fear and then re-deliver a softened version: 'oh that's not a monster, it's a shadow, moving when the light flickers, look!'

Holding and detoxifying the unwanted emotion are thus functions of the reliable 'container' – a function impeded if the mature other is, for a variety of possible reasons, also afraid, or not able to hear, or bear, the pain. For some artists with whom I spoke, art was described as providing a 'containing experience' – of holding aspects of the person which were felt to have 'nowhere else to go' and were felt to be unwanted, but nevertheless necessary, parts of one's autobiographical self. This is Sarah, for example, when I asked her what she meant by art being 'containing' after she had described it as such:

*. . . **It's** all there on a page in front of you, and you can walk away when you need a break and come back, and **it'll** all still be there, **it's** all held there and contained there for when you need **it** . . .*

(emphasis in the speech indicated in bold type)

Sarah does not elaborate on what 'it' is – but she seems to be clear that 'it', while needing to be got out, should not then evaporate into nothing, as the 'it' is something important about herself. She goes on:

There is something about art that is containing and safe. It provides you a visual vocabulary when you cannot find the words to express yourself. I think it's about the expression, being able to . . . when I lose my words, just being able to find some kind of (pause) alternative vocabulary, whether it's colours or lines . . . anything . . . that can still communicate with another person . . . em . . . it takes you out of a place of being alone, em, with feelings or thoughts . . . to this kind of shared experience with someone else . . . and once it's shared, it's less . . . for me it feels less unmanageable . . .

It's the process, you have to have the process to find meaning, going through the process kind of brings all the little strands together and then you can kind of collapse them together to make the product . . . it's much richer if you have put all the ingredients in, you've found them yourself . . . it's your journey and it's more valuable than gold. You'll be less susceptible to going back.

Looking back, I believe I was searching for something. Em, I was searching for meaning, I was searching for answers, I was searching for some kind of understanding because the not knowing was scary, was scaring me, I was out of control, I didn't know, so I was constantly producing art, er, trying to make connections, to try and gain some control of the situation and I guess art kind of gave me a little bit of that control back, like when I felt I made a link, an Aha! moment . . .

Once the 'it' is out, contained, and can be looked at or held or touched, Ehrenzweig's third stage of re-introjection can take over:

It's there now. Held for me. And you know what, sometimes it's no longer (pause) . . . quite so scary or ugly. I can . . . I need to move on . . . think about which parts of me to carry and what I now want my art to be.

(Zot Dow)

Author and therapist Julia Segal describes how once the person has experienced the sense of someone or something that has a containing function:

the capacity for thought and for tolerating bad feelings is increased . . . The ability to hold and contain sense without simply evacuating it into someone else has then been taken in. A sense of space and time is created; experience does not have to be rejected or incorporated immediately but can be held for a while. Thoughts and thinking become possible.

(1992: 122)

For another psychoanalyst and art theoretician, Kenneth Wright, art activity may be a way of the artist holding himself together in the face of early deprivation and the absence of such emotional holding. Art activity in this schema, as I explore further in the following chapter, is seen as a way of us as adults making up for a lack of interaction between infant and caregivers, a hallmark of early dysfunctional or neglectful upbringing. Certainly characteristics of such upbringings were described by a great many, although not all, of the people with whom I spoke, and are known to be associated with mental unease and ill health. Wright makes the link between such an upbringing and its later 're-visiting' through art, and describes how in art making:

> There is an emotional reaching out towards an object, with perhaps the expectation of a response; a medium that allows itself to be transformed; and a 'finding' or creating within that medium of significant forms that reveal the subject to himself.
>
> (Wright, 2009: 144)

Sometimes this interrelationship obtained through art was suggestive of a corrective emotional experience, whereby there was a sense of 'recompense'. Art practice, for some spoken of as a 'last resort', had sometimes come up with rare goods; catharsis; renewal; reliability; a sense of optimism and hope:

> *It is hard to say what art has given me . . . gives me . . . it's where I rest myself and test myself. It's always there for me, reminding me of a sense of wonder, I guess . . .*
>
> (Pippa)

But for some, art practice was described as being maintained, for a time at least, in what seemed to be an intermediate zone, before a reliable and intimate relationship with one's practice was achieved. Here art practice and its product seemed to be used as a space onto which to project, to dispel – without the artist necessarily being able to receive these projections back in digestible form. One of the most reclusive participants, Tara, spoke from the depths of such a zone:

> *By the time I was ten years old I was already engaged with the psychiatric system, given anti-depressants and benzodiazepines on a daily basis. This is when my mental illness began to unravel rapidly, and completely uncontrollably. During my adolescence and early adulthood I was subjected to endless psychotic disturbances which led me to serious self-harm, suicide attempts, social ineptitude, withdrawal and three exorcisms . . . yes literally. I wanted so desperately to purge this beast from inside of me and the demons outside who wanted to and continue to, destroy my life.*
>
> *I suppose the only concrete and meaningful activity during this time and throughout my life has been drawing and painting, writing poetry and taking photographs. I remain in the same pain and crisis as I did when I was seven . . . forty years on . . . the child within me suffers terribly, I have to try to help her as no one else can.*

She goes on to describe her art:

> *. . . the subject matter was and is at times horrific and lacking in any form of objective control, but it is what it is, it needs to be raw, honest and truthful for it to reach the subconscious. Expressive and virginal art remains my only saviour . . . as still I can find no one to truly help me.*

While it is beyond the scope of this chapter to further explore Tara's mental state, her life and how art works within it, her story does offer a glimpse of a private and pained existence in which art is clung to as a lifeline. For Tara, it seems as though the 'evacuation' stage in her art making persists, but the art work, serving as recipient of so much pain, is, perhaps, overwhelmed by it in the same way that a poorly-equipped caregiver might become overwhelmed by the projected pain in an unending infant scream. Eventually, ideally, this stage is moved beyond, when a sense of containment, of having one's pain held and modified, has been experienced. As in therapy, one of the beneficial outcomes of making art is allowing us to look upon our pain with some distance and to experience the relief of having it expressed, externalized and held outside of what sometimes feels the prison of our self. Here is the philosopher Hegel, way back in one of his lectures on Fine Art in 1835, speaking of how art liberates in this way: 'man [*sic*] is released from his immediate imprison-ment in a feeling and becomes conscious of it as something external to him, to which he must now relate himself in an ideal way' (Hegel, [1835] 1975: 49).

The Kleinian topography encompasses these themes: the need to evacuate unwanted bits of the self; the quest to see these held and contained, and experi-enced as detoxified (reactivating a primary caregiver role); the need to re-introject these parts of oneself in a move toward greater integration and wholeness, and then a move into the depressive position. Here, mourning and saying sorry, to oneself, one's objects and part objects, in a deep and profound way, is possible. Let's take a look at this theorized achievement and see what was said in the interviews of experiences which appear to allude to this.

Reparation: creative (re)solutions

The final stage in Ehrenzweig's formulation is based on Melanie Klein's formu-lation of the 'depressive position' and it is therefore worth explaining Klein's topography a bit further.[2] For Klein, the human being is from infanthood riddled with conflict and anxiety which the psyche strives to alleviate. Her theory of development departed from Freud's in presenting a more fluid, dynamic and *ongoing* process, in which we move in between two positions, the paranoid-schizoid and the depressive, throughout the lifespan, tempered by how much anxiety is being experienced and how, and by what means, we are trying to defend ourselves. It should be remembered that despite the loaded terms of 'paranoid-schizoid' and 'depressive' Klein was not referring to mental illness as such, but, usefully, how mental health and ego integration exist on a continuum. Our early experiences lay down patterns of relating and sophisticated, life-protecting ways of dealing with threat and anxiety, which are reactivated throughout our adult life.

The 'paranoid-schizoid position' refers to a collection of anxieties and defences that Klein believed were characteristic of the earliest months of life, but which continued into childhood and adulthood. In this position we deal impersonally and automatically with perceived threat and its anxiety by 'splitting off' bad feelings and projecting them out. Klein (1946) identified splitting as the most primitive of psychological defences, one which gives us a means by which to protect the self from the bad and to manage the harsh 'reality' that this bad can co-exist with the good. Klein first theorized this through depicting the pre-verbal infant as attempting to process the terrifying realization that the good mother and the bad mother were one and the same. The paranoid-schizoid position is marked by a frantic, non-reflective stance as splitting both requires and generates 'black and white' perception and an impoverished view and experience of both our inner and outer worlds. We can recognize in this activity some of the descriptions of art making in Ehrenzweig's first stage, where artists 'ejected' material, trying to rid themselves of it in the machine-gun fire of punctured canvases or in their strident, 'in your face', sometimes 'fuck you' imagery. Anxiety is kept at bay by a denial of any view that may impinge on this sense of certainty. In this state there is little room for play or symbolism as these demand the suspension of certainty and a move to reflection, to a relaxation of borders between good/bad, real/unreal, and the development of mental space. This position also involves an unconscious attack on our 'internal objects' which are constituted from people or their representations in our life – or our imagined versions of these.

It is not until the depressive position is reached (necessary for Ehrenzweig's third stage) that one moves towards the capacity for symbol formation and toleration of a sense of integration, bringing together part objects, good/bad, aspects of one's self previously kept apart. Here comes the relaxation of borders and the space this enables – and we can perhaps grasp how challenging such a relaxation might be, for someone who has travelled the corridors of trauma, blame, secrecy, deprivation and mental illness, the sum total of which demands that something in one's experience be nailed down – *be what it is, what it appears to be.*

In the depressive position, guilt is experienced in response to the attacks performed and imagined in the prior paranoid-schizoid position. Concern arises, and reparation is felt to be needed and possible. This may be reparation to others, 'bits' of others, or indeed to ourselves, victim to self-chastisement, persecution and hate that we have been made to feel towards ourselves, a hatred sometimes deeply rooted in our infant experiences. The depressive position is marked by a mental slowing down, and an inevitable mourning, as the 'simple' certainty of black/white, hate/love, idolization/denigration is lost. This makes way for an altogether more complex, nuanced and necessarily painful perception of both inner and outer worlds, where anxiety is *tolerated*. Identity takes on yet another form – that of survivor, perhaps, as the long view holds out a landscape in which to reposition ourselves. In this landscape insight is gained not only into one's mental states, but one's history, the actions of others, where blame should fall, but also, importantly, where gratitude should be apportioned; it is a stage of moral reckoning. Klein's model, and its development through object relations psychoanalysis more broadly, has been pointed to as one that suggests an innate relatedness in the human being, a model through which to 'explain complex configurations of moral feeling, both within individuals and in societies' (Rustin, 2001: 190).

Achievement and completion, both in the psychic and artistic sense, usher in new means of being in the world. Charlie Devus, who describes himself as a story-telling artist, says this:

I have tried to do everything to avoid talking about myself, I have used metaphors to get around the pain of my own life . . . but gradually as I achieve more, as I complete more, I am able to talk about my own life . . . although I think I need to do that . . . but I think a lot of it has been an attempt to deal with my life without actually having to look at the reality of it . . . it was very painful . . . (pause) when you have suffered abuse as a child and your main abuser is your mother, who was a highly intelligent, highly educated, highly articulate, manipulator . . . it's very difficult to have a voice, because you simply aren't believed, in fact you don't believe it yourself . . .

For Martha, the process of working on an artistic project begins with making something grow out of '*all that mess and emotional chaos*' and watching how:

. . . these feelings that I had were coming out through print-making techniques and the drawings I was doing without me really planning it.

This process then reaches a point of resolution:

But the really sort of fundamental therapeutic side where it [art practice] is taking a feeling or a traumatic experience or something like that, the difficult things you have . . . and working that through into a final set of creative solutions . . .

Regardless of the extent to which we buy into the Kleinian formulation, we can recognize characteristics inherent in this schema which relate to a concept of mental health/illness. Feelings of anxiety and persecution lead to a 'locking down' of our ability to consider the other; to tolerate ambivalence and ambiguity. They lead to us lashing out as we try to rid ourselves of the awfulness we are experiencing. They summon a depleted view of the world and ourselves, weighed down as we are by the 'badness' of everything, as a result of us having stripped it of any good in our human attempt to preserve, separately, whatever good there might be, and thus keep some sanity and order in our worlds. The idolized good, in turn, is unsustainable, attached to objects which cannot bear the weight of so much expectation, the proverbial placing of all our eggs in one basket. The depressive position, too, we may recognize; that easing of the mind, where we catch a glimpse of something beyond; where we realize that all is not that bad, but neither is our 'prized' object – be it art, a significant other, a new therapy, a new identity – infallible, and we have to acknowledge its limitations. There is a fluidity to our feelings as we accept that we cannot and do not *know*. And there is the possibility of repair. We set about the world again with whatever tools we have – missing the certainty of aggressive attack, but charged instead with the human compulsion to repair and build. Some of our resolutions are creative; some are a revisiting of old solutions – they mostly all have a life-preserving, life-enhancing aim. Here is Chloe Shalini:

For some years a lot of my paintings concerned my emotional state. I'm relieved to say . . . I am now entering a very different stage in my development. I no longer need to paint my anguish and violation . . . Although I no longer seem to need to paint my emotions I am certainly painting my spiritual journey.

And Adena suggested that, slowly, '*it [the art] becomes less about pain and blame*'.

Many of the participants spoke about this 'coming to terms' as an important part of their lives. There were features of it which echo those of the depressive position, such as acceptance, forgiveness and gratitude. The integration experienced after the evacuation and re-integration heralded a new sense of coherence; in one's art and one's identity, but particularly in how the two 'worked' together. There was a new sense verbalized, of 'who I am' *vis-à-vis* my illness; my art; and the experiences which caused me damage:

> *. . . I am predisposed to see the world in very black and white terms, and I wonder and hope that I might find a more integrated whole.*
>
> (Crystal)

> *Me and bipolar are one and the same, they're intrinsically linked and I wouldn't be me without it.*
>
> (Jasmine)

> *I think my body will always be present in the art, I mean even when I'm making work on other bodies I still use the camera and it's my body working the camera so I think all the time . . . the medium that I happen to be using . . . I think the body will always be present, I think even when I create paintings or I'm working with other materials I still feel it's the body that's my common denominator. I feel very loyal to it as well you know it's the thing that's been my greatest demon but is also a huge asset so really the two, er . . . actually I think it will always be from the body I mean this association, this illness has been with me since I was very young so I know it better than anything else and that's the thing that's become a rich pool of information for me and I don't feel like I've even got very far into it yet . . .*
>
> (Liz Atkin)

The coming to terms with one's 'demons and assets', the creative resolution, was expressed, but was also *experienced* through the work itself. Here is Liz Atkin again, on her forthcoming exhibition in which she displays her illness in her work for the first time:

> *And so it's a bold move to speak about my illness but one that I feel very comfortable with, in fact it feels quite empowering to be able to say the truth and for that truth to be out there. It feels like the right time, I'm in a comfortable place in my life, I feel secure, and yeah, I'm trusting that it's a good thing to do, and having a conversation with someone like you as well (laughs) and being able to talk to a stranger more openly about it, it feels to me like something quite significant and it feels like the right time.*

For some of the people with whom I spoke, implicated in this journey towards a creative resolution was, in their words, a moral reckoning; a taking and giving of an account of one's self (Butler, 2005). Through an art practice which was raw with confrontations of one's 'demons and assets'; which 'aligned itself' with the history of an illness and which required disclosure of a past as well as offering a propelling forward, a kind of 'puncturing' seems to have taken place for some, and a reading, through this, of one's moral compass. This, evoking Badiou (2001), acted as a 'truth event' – where there was movement in a situation from the known to the unknown, and in this disturbance, a propelling into a new ontological state. The ethic of a truth, for Badiou, requires fidelity to the consequences of such an event – acting upon the fresh awareness, and indeed some individuals spoke of such a 'no going back'. The insights, disturbances and demands of their art practice had led to a reconfiguration of different areas of their life and their stance towards others.

This, along with the other processes and challenges described in this chapter, will be familiar to professionals working within a psychodynamic paradigm, and to those who are familiar with the many claims that narrative identity is a process of reordering and sifting, building and connecting. What is noteworthy here is that in these narratives, moves towards order, integration and reparation were happened upon autonomously; a difference, perhaps crucial, for some of these individuals. The agency and the creativity in finding a non-verbal, non-lexical means by which to move forward suggests that people who have not engaged in therapy can, and often do, find other ways of addressing their past, their illnesses and a narrative through which to move on.

It is also important to keep in mind the nature of some of the illnesses held within this group of narrators. Illnesses which in some cases are enduring; subject to remission and then re-ignition; needing for their management, vigilance, insight, sheer perseverance and resilience. Living with some of these histories, traumas and illnesses is a lifetime existential project, one which, if you have few words with which to say it, but some forms with which to show it, is best managed through an ongoing creative and analytic project.

Notes

1 This ability of art making to '*open cans of worms*', as more than one participant put it, has also been the subject of reports by art therapists who have expressed concern regarding Arts in Health projects which ask people to explore emotional issues, without the supervisory, ethical and theoretical frameworks on which art therapists base their working practice (Angus, 2002).

2 Readers wishing to look further into Kleinian and object relations theory of art are referred to Glover (2009) and Gosso (2004).

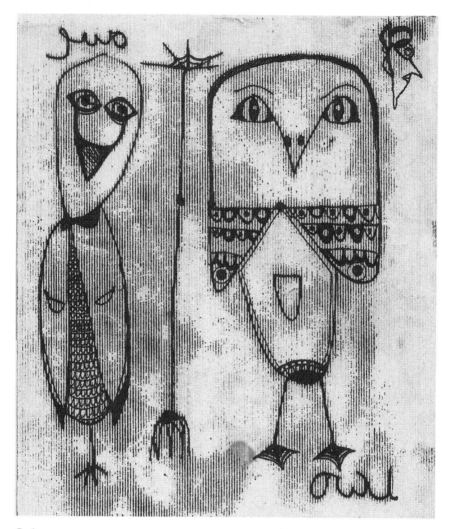

Owls

6 Mirrors and connection

> Imagination is what enables us to cross the empty spaces between ourselves and those we have called 'others'.
>
> (Maxine Greene, 1995)

This chapter turns our attention to a further theme distinct in the narratives of the art makers who spoke to me – that of *connection*. Whilst it is a truism that 'art connects', something I heard tell frequently, I wanted to probe further into what was meant by this and to look at what sorts of experiences lay behind this spoken of '*sense of connection*'. I also wanted to explore the possible meanings of such highly valued experiences, for what they might tell us about the interface of art and mental wellbeing.

In this chapter I draw again on selected psychoanalytic theory, using it to help further an understanding of the role of connection through art making. I draw on concepts which spring from the British Object Relations tradition – concepts such as mirroring, attunement and attachment, all of which speak of a fundamental human need to be seen and to be in resonant connection with other(s). I will begin by looking at what people said about discovering a connection with themselves – a theme that has already breathed through the previous two chapters and is one that seems to hold a key to some of the therapeutic punch of making art. I then return to a concern from Chapter 3, where I looked to the narratives to trace how art makers with mental health difficulties moved into a more mainstream art practice, and further explore what people told me about how art helped forged a connection to others.

Connecting within: discovery and memory

> *Art brings me into contact with sides of my personality that are surprising, and it's a journey . . . an exploration that is exciting. It creates better understanding and connection to people and the world around me. It's a discovery as well as a memory.*
>
> (Yelena)

The experience of mental illness has often been described as alienating; an individual can become a foreigner in her own skin, not recognizing her ways of thinking or behaving. An episode of mental illness can almost literally knock us off our feet – disrupting our sense of continuity, and making us sceptical about who we thought we were. Such identity vertigo makes our previous knowledge of ourselves and others seem fickle, and relating to either becomes difficult. As Baldwin (2005) suggests, the experiences accompanying serious mental illness threaten narrative agency, continuity and coherence and at such times a person may become highly susceptible to the medical mental illness narrative. That narrative, embedded within a mental health culture which Repper and Perkins (2003) amongst others see as pessimistic and disempowering, disrupts the ability to maintain or create a personal story which is continuous and which holds resonant connections with one's life experiences. '*Finding ways back, back to me*', *as* Zot Dow put it, becomes an important process within each person's road map through illness. Basset and Stickley draw our attention to the skills of living that people with experiences of mental illness thus oftentimes acquire, observing that:

> If anybody can teach us about how to live in our modern, or postmodern world, it is people who have struggled with the complexities of existence and found their own unique ways of surviving, learning and moving on.
>
> (2010: 1)

In Chapters 4 and 5 I talked about the experience of identity fragmentation that is so often reported by sufferers of mental illness. In numerous texts and testimony people have reported feeling as though they were falling apart; in bits; disconnected; and a rich seam of narrative studies in health has shown how people try to cope with these dissonant experiences.[1] Arthur Frank (1995), as I have described in Chapter 4, shows how stories of journeys through illness are sometimes framed as 'chaos narrative', where there is no respite; 'restitution narrative', where there is a belief in going back to an 'old self'; or 'quest narrative', where individuals do not refer to going back to a pre-illness identity, but rather, feel that their illness is an integral part of themselves. They would move ahead *with* it; managing, modifying, understanding the illness and themselves in relation to it.

> What is quested for may never be wholly clear, but the quest is defined by the ill person's belief that something is to be gained through the experience.
>
> (Frank, 1995: 115)

Almost all the narratives I looked at for this book rested on a form of this latter 'quest narrative'. It was as part of this quest narrative that there emerged descriptions of how art was instrumental in helping people connect with a previously fragmented part of themselves in order to move on. As the extract from Yelena's narrative at the start of this section described, echoing Ricoeur (1970) once more, art seems to offer an exploration which is both *discovery and memory*; a process of striking out ahead *and* looking back, bringing both together in the art making.

There were a great many instances of people describing how through their art they were able to make connections. These were sometimes between an image and what lay behind it, as mentioned in the previous chapter, and between an experience and an image, as mentioned in Chapter 4. But there were also numerous references to making connections with other parts of oneself, or other personalities. In the more extreme instances, as with artists who were diagnosed with Dissociative Identity Disorder (DID), this was spoken of as a particularly powerful experience. Harli Tree, an artist diagnosed with DID, talks here about how art gave her access to other 'selves':

> *[art gives me an] insight because then I know how they [the other parts] are feeling. I didn't know how many parts there were but there has been a painting . . . and you will notice that there is a difference in one of the first paintings to one of the recent paintings . . . that there is another part. So where there were eight parts, that includes me in the eight, there are now nine . . . There are younger parts that don't talk. So their painting, if they paint, then that is their voice.*

Whilst it is beyond the scope of this chapter or indeed this book to look in more detail at the fascinating but troubling experience of being an artist diagnosed with DID, Harli Tree's narrative describes an intense personal experience of connection with 'other parts' which has been possible only through her own, accelerating practice of making art. As some 'parts' have no verbal ability and can only tell their story – in some cases quite a traumatic one – through painting, this medium has become crucial in Harli Tree's gaining of knowledge about her past and insight into her condition: '*So if a part gets distressed or if they want to say something, artwork will be done.*'

Other artists too spoke about this sense of connecting with parts of themselves, claiming that this sense of connection both aided, and was part of, their journey through mental illness. As Tam put it, '*I need to know the "me" that I'm taking with me through all this [hands circling the head] and art is a tool in that . . .*'

Charlie Devus spoke of coming to know and integrate the different ethnicities in his family history which he found to be an important element in his gradual location of himself. They made themselves 'known' through his art making:

> *. . . I realize I've split into about seven different ethnicities because my father was . . . my grandfather was German apparently with some quite right wing sympathies during the war when he came from America. My grandmother was Jewish but she didn't even know it, my maternal grandmother. My grandfather was descended from Irish convicts and Danes as well and there are Welsh socialists and Scots in there and I notice that I, having found finally the last element of all this, or at least I thought it was the last element, I can now look at seven different aspects of my persona . . . seeing how they come out in different facets of my art.*

And Chloe Shalini found that art making helps her connect with both negative and positive parts of herself, art acting as a check and balance in her perspective of herself as a person:

> *. . . the best thing about it [art] is it's a means of communication even if it's just to yourself of what is within you, whatever that may be, it doesn't have to be a negative thing. For me at the*

moment the nice thing is that I am able to . . . I feel like I am bringing out positive things. Or the intention is rather to bring out positive things onto a canvas or a paper rather than to illustrate some sort of distress . . . (pause) . . . there is a kind of universal unity sort of thing.

Kayleigh offered a characteristically humorous analogy:

I get it . . . (pause) . . . it's not like I've 'found me' [makes scare marks] through art – but it is a bit like holding up a mirror time and again and, you know, sometimes you see the zits, sometimes you see the nice bits. Sometimes the zits matter and you work on that. Other times, what matters (pause) . . . is all the fine points. Sometimes too, you think: Oh My God! Is that me, like, REALLY?

In Chapter 4 I looked at how accessing experience and memories and externalizing these was felt to be valuable. From people's testimony it would seem that art making aids a connection with oneself which may be experienced as facilitating insight and fuelling the journey on which each person feels herself to be. It offers a journey of both memory and discovery, one which includes, for some, a better understanding of the damaging effects of one's own limiting beliefs about illness, trauma and their wake. Here is Kayleigh again:

. . . I simply did not KNOW how small I thought myself to be . . . until I painted it . . . this tiny, formless person, floating around, no . . . substance . . . easily . . . (pause) . . . battered . . .

The early Greek exhortation at Delphi to 'Know Thyself' did not come with an accompanying inscribed instruction manual. And while the aphorism has resounded compellingly throughout the centuries since, the object of knowledge has been through convoluted definitions with our understanding of it in constant flux. Yet the human drive to understand one's self better has far from abated. And for some, experiences of disruption, trauma, illness and hurt make this drive the more urgent as attempts are made to square the circle of biographical disruption (Bury, 1982, 1991) and come to grips with why stuff happens in the way it does and what on earth it might mean.

Whilst the concept of self that is endorsed by the phenomenological tradition may not be generalized outside Western developed cultural contexts, within this context waves of both collective and individual 'self-searching' have dotted contemporary history, as shortcomings of each economic and political system lead to renewed interest in alternative ways of living, and hence of being. A sustained art practice seems, for some, to offer a means, at the very least, to see things about one's self differently. It offers a 'tool for life' – one which can be reliably looked to not only for understanding a past and an illness, but for gaining a self-understanding on an ongoing basis:[2]

I've got to grips with the illness myself, independently, and now my understanding of it and my . . . erm . . . my art work is closely linked to how I am keeping well and . . . [it] is like

*a daily reprieve for me. I have a way to manage it and cope with it and handle it which makes
. . . has made me well and keeps me well.*

(Jil)

*. . . But for me the crucial thing is that when you make art . . . you can get emotions out
that you're too scared of facing and putting words to. You can just look at them as a form
and when you look at them they may mean something different to what they mean to me. So
I also don't have to be too exposing in the stuff that I put out but I understand what it means
to me.*

(Eilish)

Art therapist Martina Thomson, drawing on Basch's (1981) idea of 'selfing', put
it like this:

> As the body, the organism, is continually modified by its interaction with the
> environment, by an ongoing process of exchange between inner and outer, so
> is the self. When we speak of the self we are referring to a process and not an
> entity. 'Selfing' would more aptly describe it.

(Thomson, 1989: 48)

This notion of 'selfing' – with the continuous tense suggesting both the unremit-
tingness, and the 'now', of the project – came through in people's narratives. It is
a project that carries particular weight and meaning for those who have
experienced the ravages of the self that are wrought by mental illness and our
sometimes less than sensitive ways of helping people through it. But the project of
selfing is inevitably performed *in dialogue* with an outside, with an other. Here is
Andrew Locke, a multimedia artist who uses his art to explore his experiences with
schizophrenia, dance, music and synaesthesia:

*[it's] almost like the resolution to a problem. Going out of oneself in order to create something
that will make you feel more together. I would call this 'a creative flight' . . .*

In the Winnicottian scheme of things alluded to by Thomson, there is an interplay between our inner world and the outer; between a 'me' and the environment
– an interplay which is our first challenge as infants. Busy with negotiating the
boundaries of me/not me, we move beyond a feeling of complete merger with a
primary caregiver, and make use of the 'transitional object' – the iconic comfort
blanket of our babyhood. Working the challenges and rewards of the 'potential
space' (Winnicott, 1971), where space is neither entirely of the external world nor
entirely of one's inner world, we breathe in a pliable space where the lack of
demarcation and territorial rules offers at least a temporary sense of freedom and
play. It is a space of shared warmth and creation for both the primary caregiver
and the infant; an intermediate area of experience. And it is here that patterns are
laid down for 'intense experiencing that belongs to the arts and to religion and to
imaginative living, and to creative scientific work' (Winnicott, 1971: 10). Does art

making offer us, as adults, a means of experimenting with this remembered or desired interplay in such an accommodating space? Dialogue indeed formed the backdrop of many of the experiences of making art that were described; a dialogue between, but also situated in, an intermediate area, a liminal space between 'me/not me'; between art and life; between illness and health and between illness and art. Townsend (2013: 181) describes how in the fleeting moments in the creation of art works, 'there is no distinction between the me and the not-me. Inside and outside not only coincide, they cannot be distinguished.'

And whilst the dialogue was spun through a connection with oneself that art making seemed to facilitate, and this bringing together of the outside and the in, it was also spun in connection with others. It is to this strand of the narrative that I now turn.

Connecting with out: being seen, disclosing and displaying

In Chapter 3, I traced how people with a passion for art making and experiences of mental health difficulties had made transitions into an art practice. I listened to what they said about what was in place for them to formalize an art practice, for them to move out of their initial space and place of art making, and heard them speak of how accessible, or not, opportunities beyond this were. In speaking about the changing face of their art activity, participants told me a lot about their experiences of connection to other people, and how art practice, as observed by Parr (2012: 8), can be 'an important "stepping stone" into wider social geographies'. In this section I go back to the narratives to hear what was said about the particular experience of connection to *others*, and why it was felt to be of such significance.

It has long been established that one of the greatest determinants of health is the extent to which we are socially connected (Marmot and Wilkinson, 2005). A large body of work in the social sciences attributes a positive value to participation and identifies links between subjective feelings of wellbeing and companionship (see *inter alia* Lane, 2000). Psychological functioning is intrinsically bound with how we relate to others, and mental wellbeing is generally regarded as being at least to some extent dependent on us having satisfactory levels of connection with other people and with a world outside of our own. Psychoanalyst and philosopher Erich Fromm, in his still highly popular book *The Sane Society*, argued that the sense of identity that is the very touchstone of sanity was dependent on a sense of belonging forged in relation to others. Theories and explorations spanning sociology, anthropology, psychology and psychiatry offer up sophisticated ways of looking at how we connect, stay connected and how our connections impact on our mental and physical health – pleading, perhaps, for an integrated approach (Berkman *et al.*, 2000).

That said, we should remain sceptical of how in our current cultural and political climate the promoting of relationships, community, team working and so on is relentless, as part of a discourse that allows the state and welfare provision to be in slow but steady retreat. It is a discourse that allows little wriggle room for those who may wish to live otherwise. It is also a discourse that is confusing; simultaneously warning of the perils of isolation *and* touting independence.

A plethora of websites, for example, giving advice on better mental health recommend belonging to support groups, strengthening one's networks and maintaining friendship groups. The New Economics Foundation's project *Five Ways to Well-Being* concluded that five simple steps incorporated into daily life can fortify mental health – top of the list: 'Connect: Developing relationships enriches life and brings support'. A self-help for depression website places the directive 'cultivate supportive relationships' at the very top of its list of self-help tips. And within this discourse of the relational it is easy to see how, yet again, the person not conforming to, or not able to buy into this zeitgeist of collective recovery, may experience the guilt, the shame or the burden of not doing the 'right' thing to help themselves. While the narratives I gathered almost unequivocally favoured the power of connecting with others, such a tension of discourse must be held in mind when looking at narrative in the area of mental health; after all, those in favour of solitude and privacy would clearly be less likely to want to speak with me.

Since the sociologist Émile Durkheim in the 1890s first claimed that the structure of society had a strong bearing on psychological health, research within psychiatry and the social sciences more broadly has been exploring the impact of the social context on mental wellbeing.[3] The concept of 'social capital' has latterly been embraced as a possible means by which to explain some of the differences in health that are found between places or between groups of people, to predict vulnerability and prevalence of mental illness (McKenzie and Harpham, 2006; Morgan and Swann, 2004), and to describe the social benefits of arts engagement (White 2006, 2009; Eames, 2003). Indeed some disorders and much distress are characterized by extreme withdrawal, lack of social functioning and almost phobic reactions to any engagement with the social world. A notable share of first person narrative of illness literature echoes Guarneri's (2007) axiom that 'the "I" in illness is isolation, and the crucial letters in wellness are "we"'. In Chapter 3 I looked at how working with and through others was described as an important means by which people moved out of a clinical context and mindset of 'ill' and into a more agentic artistic being and identity. This movement was engendered, it would seem, through both the bonding (connecting with others within one's milieu) and bridging (connecting with others outside of one's immediate milieu) forms of social capital, enabling people to connect; share; pool resources and benefit from a strength drawn from numbers, 'we-ness' and solidarity of cause. The discourse of social connectedness within health and recovery literature and policy (Secker *et al.*, 2007) is pervasive – appearing often under the more socio-economically resonant term 'social inclusion' – and it would seem irrefutable that participation in arts activity can strengthen ties within groups and communities and enhance people's sense of civic belonging (Kelaher *et al.*, 2013). My intention in this part of this chapter is not to question this outcome, but to look more closely at this narrated experience of connectedness and discuss how this might be linked to wellbeing.

People in this book often referred to a 'social' aspect of making art, describing art making's ability to lift you *out* of your 'self' as being importantly linked to an improved sense of wellbeing and enhanced self-esteem (Geddes, 2004). As quipped by Jil, '*I'll get out of bed for art . . .*'

Here is Sue, followed by Catherine:

> *. . . it boosts my self-esteem when people like my work, it helps me to push all these problems away and say no, I'm not going to be treated like that . . . I'm not going to let anyone treat me like that, I am a creative person, and I am worth something . . .*

> *. . . that thing of being part of a group has been really good for me . . . That's one of the things that comes from being involved with the arts, being part of a group, who are working on something. It has helped me think more about where I live, I go out and photograph things nearby, I get involved with local groups and that's all because I want to be involved in creative activities.*

It has been noted (see *inter alia* Stickley, 2012) that in trying to evaluate the impact of arts activity in mental health, it is very hard to extricate the therapeutic in the making from that in the social; even more so if we frame art making as inevitably being a connection with an other, in dialogue, as mentioned above. There were traces of narrative which clearly alluded to the social capital and sense of wellbeing generated through the practice of making; but the making seemed tightly woven with embodied and personal experiences of disclosing, sharing, and displaying. People spoke of the networks, friendships and the solidarity which often came with them 'coming out' as having a mental illness, and how displaying their work gave them immense boosts of self-confidence, even euphoria. Sarah was one of several who had taken a carefully considered decision about disclosure in her artwork and display:

> *I was really cautious to begin with, really, really cautious . . . I was aware that I was going to be doing something a bit controversial but then I think I just got a bit rebellious as well because I thought, if someone has a sore leg they can talk about their sore leg and it's absolutely fine. If someone has mental health problems, why is there such a stigma around it? Why can't they talk about this also? I just felt rebellious and thought well I'm just going to talk about it because if I talk about it then maybe someone else will talk about it.*

The experience of both disclosure and display within spaces felt to be safe and containing was highly valued as an important step towards inclusion in a wider community, one that offered a sense of 'belonging'. Yet as pointed out by Parr (2012: 4), some such opportunities may provide 'bonding and not necessarily bridging social capital for participants' with more dense ties being made between members of a particular group whose members are joined by a shared sense of belonging and identity – while connection with the wider community remains limited. This limited opportunity to develop social capital may be 'postponing' the inevitable experience of stigma and exclusion which accompanies exposure and circulation in the wider community. Nevertheless, bonding within containing groups that knew 'the shorthand' of one's artist practice was deemed to offer an important time and space for self-development in which resilience could be built; resilience that would help with later, wider exposure. Here is Tam:

> *These are people who I know I can . . . (pause) I can 'cut to the chase' with. They know what I'm talking about, in my art, they know the shorthand, when I talk about it . . . I don't need to back-pedal and explain stuff around mental illness, they get it, and so . . . I get room, to move on in my thinking, all the time, within this group . . . and I feel like I am practising, no, not practising, kind of learning, skills, confidence, getting my armour together (laughs) for challenges ahead, places where maybe people don't 'get it' quite so well . . .*

As we saw in Chapter 3, the trajectory on and beyond such projects and groups was not always smooth. How one moved on from the initial disclosure through one's art, its display and the 'safety' of the group and how one used newly gained or recovered confidence and life skills was an experience often marred with difficulty. For some, a decision was made to *not* venture beyond what had become a very private art practice. Amongst the people with whom I spoke there were a small number whose domain of art practice had remained private, asserting that it was only in this way that relief from pain was to be found. Poonam was one artist who felt little need to go beyond her private practice, as her practice as it was gave her a connection to something beyond herself – a 'beyonding' which had spiritual connotations and was felt to powerfully impact on her wellbeing:

> *It [art making] allows me to 'out' thoughts and feelings. Sometimes I get so absorbed I forget about my anxieties. I also feel connected to a lineage that's beyond my situational circumstance – a higher self of some kind . . . This other, helps me . . . (pause) I can't explain it, without it sounding religious. It's not like that. It's a guiding light, kind. And I am connected with it through making art.*

Tara, whom readers may recall from the previous chapter, was another artist whose solitary way of life and art making was important to her. She described how she had made regular forays into the 'world' but had come back to her reclusive way of life:

> *I realized in my twenties that although I was incredibly 'mad', I was also extremely bright and creative. I tried many different outlets for my creative urges including relationships, motherhood and academia, and although I achieved much success in all these areas my mental illness was always beside me making everything even more difficult, more random, more irregular. Having nervous, mental breakdowns approximately every two to three years since childhood to present day has charred my existence then and now beyond belief. My role as mother, daughter and student has had to be put on hold so many times during breakdowns and the recovery processes. Yet I fought and continue to fight on, through resistance, resentment and deep emotional scarring I continue the battle.*

So here I am now, forty-seven years old, with a new body of work, a recluse. Completely socially isolated, no friends; well versed in psychiatry and its limitations.

The piece of writing in its entirety reads as painful testament, reminding us again of the darkness and struggle which is part of the reality of mental illness. It is beyond the scope of this chapter to do justice to Tara's mental state and how art works within it; neither do I have access to a fuller picture of her to enable us both to elaborate on this. Suffice to say at this point that for some, the relief offered by an art practice resides *precisely* in it being private. From Tara's testimony, it is only in such privacy, even isolation, that her art making can function to offer her relief. It is important, then, that Arts in Health interventions acknowledge the different modalities of art engagement, and address the need of people to connect, but also respect their need to *disconnect* at times – without the risk of them being further pathologized. In making art and experiencing it as therapeutic, the private and the social both play a part, sometimes at different points in the artist's journey.

In further considering the private and the social, the inner and outer, and connections with others, I turn to the experience of *being seen*, disclosing and displaying.

Experiences of feeling invisible emerged powerfully across the interviews. Such poignant descriptions spoke of an isolated, isolating negation of self, identity, even of humanness, a sense less dehumanizing than *unhumanizing*. Such experiences lay beyond voicelessness, in an even more fundamentally hollow zone of not being seen, and of eventually questioning one's very existence. For most who referred to such an experience, it was hard for them to pin down whether this painful existential state was rooted in their early years, in trauma, in its aftermath, as part of the development of mental illness, or as a by-product, again, of dehumanizing systems and the alienating and discriminatory effects of social stigma. Paul, for example, was amongst several people who spoke of invisibility as being part of their earliest memories:

> *I don't recall her [mother] really **seeing** me . . . I can't (pause) I can't remember her eyes actually engaging . . . and then, at the same time, being invisible was the safest way to be, around her . . . so maybe I opted for that . . . being invisible.*

For some, traumatic early years experiences had activated self-preservation 'skills' of dissociation (Freyd *et al.*, 2005), where we hold parts of our experience as a 'foreign body' within ourselves. This phenomenon was first conjectured by Josef Breuer and Sigmund Freud in their 'Studies on hysteria' in 1895: 'the psychical trauma or more precisely the memory of the trauma acts like a foreign body which long after its entry must continue to be regarded as an agent that is still at work . . .' (Breuer and Freud, 1955: 6). This was echoed, sometimes very movingly, in hesitant narrative extracts that alluded to, in Birdy's words, '*something in me . . . of me, that I've never got to know . . . don't want to know. It's part of me but not. It makes trouble.*' In others, a complicated relationship with being seen had emerged from a habitual hiding from a volatile caregiver. Here is Eilish:

I was seen a lot . . . I tried to make myself even less seen, 'cause every time I was seen I was in trouble . . . so my desire for invisibility . . . made the paradox come true that I was permanently visible . . .

And Leonne describes moving towards greater visibility through the safety of her painting:

I would try and make myself invisible . . . I thought I could magic it up! It would protect me from it [the abuse]. Then you figure it out later . . . that people really do just look through you 'cause you've made yourself . . . a nothing. Painting . . . I could be a something again, find a way to put myself forward, show who I was. So I wanted to be seen then, and painting, then showing my stuff, made me . . . visible. Seen through showing . . . I like that!

For some artists, like Pippa, coming to be seen was intrinsically bound with disclosing:

I felt that people were looking at my painting, seeing the colours, and maybe for the first time seeing me; because I am those colours. And in them, well they say it. The darkness, the light, the comings and goings of tones. So it was out there, and then I could say . . . also tell it, about the illness . . . and it was part of the same story, but people could maybe see it more clearly, rather than just put their own meanings into what it is to be bipolar . . .

And Sarah:

Yeh, I've had some of the people's responses, [to her exhibition] they've . . . some people especially with my most recent screen prints, they've asked me what they've been about and I've never really had that because my art work's always been so private . . . but in saying that it [disclosing] was one of the best things I ever did, because I had an exhibition, and I had to exhibit this particular screen print and some others and I had to write an artist's statement and I was very, very honest in what I wrote and I was expecting people to be quite negative and I dunno, just to judge me somehow. But I got a really positive response and I was told that it was very brave of me and bold and I received lots of really encouraging emails. It just really inspired me to keep going and that what I was doing was right.

Being seen and having a sense of being recognized is an important first stage to disclosing and to announcing the 'I am'. This 'I am' pulls in its bow wave possibilities for sharpened agency and empowerment. But why is the inscrutable experience of being seen so important that it emerges time and again? For many psychoanalytic thinkers, infant experiences of being seen in the reflection of the caregiver's eyes are crucial for our development. For Winnicott (1971), the mother's face is the child's first mirror, and it is through containment and the 'reverie' of maternal care (Bion, 1962a) that the 'me' and 'not/me' boundaries between the self and other are said to be defined. In this stage of seeing one's self reflected back, patterns of relating to others and to ourselves are internalized. For Sue Gerhardt, psychoanalytic psychotherapist and early child development specialist: 'There is a basic alchemy at work in human relationships. The attention that parents give their baby is spun, not into gold, but into the baby's own capacity to pay attention to himself' (Gerhardt, 2010: 76).

Being seen, in turn, we see and value ourselves; 'paradoxically, "I-ness" is made possible by the other' (Ogden, 1992: 209). In the best of scenarios, during what Mahler (1968) called 'the symbiotic phase', there is, in Winnicott's terms, a 'good-enough' fit between the infant and the caregiver. The caregiver is able to confer a sense of wellbeing on the infant through selective, intuitive responses and sensitive attunement (Stern, 1985), what Bersani called 'a reciprocal attention to the other's becoming' (Bersani and Phillips, 2008: 123). In the rapidly expanding field of neuroscience which is beginning to share startling insights with psychoanalytic psychology we know that cued behaviour – anticipating and responding – helps the brain activate previously dormant neural pathways, communication itself enabling infant human development (Rilling *et al.*, 2002; Grossmann *et al.*, 2010).

Such a sense, developed through positive interaction, lays the foundation of the Winnicottian, 'true self'. This 'true self' does not refer to a core, pre-existent self, but rather, to a core strength and uniqueness that enables one to trust in one's own creation of reality. Fonagy and Bateman (2007: 90) draw on Winnicott, to describe it thus:

> We speculate that when a child does not have the opportunity to develop a self-representation through the caregiver's mirroring, he internalizes the non-contingent image of the caregiver as part of his self-representation (Winnicott, 1956). We have called this discontinuity within the self the 'alien self'.

The attending caregiver, by presenting him/herself and regularly relieving the infant's distress, conveys the 'illusion that there is an external reality [that] corresponds to his own capacity to create' (Winnicott, 1953: 95). The sense that results, of being able to create and recreate, forms the basis of our ability to play and hence, of our creative potential. In being seen, in being held, we become – and in becoming we can play and create. Much of the psychoanalytic writing on mirroring and attunement has been criticized for idealizing this maternal role, and despite references in this text as in others to the 'primary caregiver', there remains the inevitable trace of gender assumptions. It is useful then to heed the words of psychoanalyst Christopher Bollas (1987: 14) who suggests that 'the mother of early infancy is less significant and identifiable as an object than as a process that is identified with cumulative internal and external transformations'. This idea of 'process' is key. Not only for removing the Mother *per se*, from the interaction that is being described between inner and outer, but for centring our attention more acutely on the developmental course in which so much is at stake in terms of learning, identity, play and, later, aesthetic engagement.

This dialectic of being seen for who we feel ourselves to be, and, in turn, this being seen inspiring further openness and creating, was an ebb and flow suggested in many of the narratives. Indeed references to finding oneself, or gripping, however fleetingly, to a more congruent sense of 'me', have been mentioned in the two preceding chapters. Part of a desire to piece together a sense of self shattered by mental illness, this wish may also hark back to the injury of having adopted a 'false self' through experiencing trauma, neglect or unreliable, chaotic relating at the hands of adults who failed to adequately 'see' an infant. This may have been further compounded by the teachers who failed to see the child; the doctors who failed to see the person; the institutional practices that failed to see the human being – and so on, as is the watermark of experience in so many lives in which mental unease develops. Eilish recounts how:

> *. . . as soon as I started my hospital treatment as an outpatient, I now understand, that unless I was physically speaking or being seen, I felt invisible.*

The establishment of a false self was linked by Winnicott to psychological disturbance. He maintained that the imposition of such a self 'is associated with the idea that nothing really matters and that life is not worth living' (1991: 65), for nothing quite rings 'true' or is experienced, at a deep and fundamental human level, as resonating with the self. The converse, 'a life worth living', has been noted as an important factor in at least one study of the arts in mental health (Spandler *et al.*, 2007), and indeed, throughout the narratives of artists in this book there were references to art 'making life worth living' or, as Tam put it, giving '*me a reason to be . . . when I'm making art, I come alive . . .*'

Sarah graphically describes the experience, common to many people with whom I spoke, of the chronic emptiness during an episode of illness. It is a salutary reminder of the experiences endured regularly, by many:

> *I don't think. I don't feel that I feel anything. That's the nightmare. I have a kind of, I call it a psychotic whisper. It is part of my mind that is going on all the time and although I feel very, very empty . . . I feel very empty and I can't process anything and I become very indifferent. Traditionally I would withdraw and not answer the phone and just lie really. So yes it's a huge feeling of emptiness and accompanied by the feeling of being very bad for being empty. In fact I have gone through phases where I've believed I was evil, which is an odd one because I haven't really been religious. I am not but I wasn't then but I definitely have decided I was evil. Yes, it's that, it's a huge feeling of emptiness and indifference.*

For some artists, art making was able – in a way not found through any other therapeutic, medical, leisure or cultural activity – to, as Zot Dow put it: '*rush blood into the veins . . . make me feel SOMETHING . . .*'. Some even spoke of '*only feeling truly alive*' when they painted, or made their art:

> *I come alive. I believe I am here. I am seen.*
>
> (Zot Dow)

The establishment of a false, compliant self forecloses on an important two-way communicative process, what psychoanalyst and attachment theorist Peter Fonagy has suggested is an evolutionarily protected epistemic superhighway for knowledge acquisition. This open-channelled communication process is built in infancy through ostensive communication cues such as eye contact; turn-taking contingent reactivity; and the use of special vocal tones by the primary caregiver, sometimes called 'motherese' – in other words, a communicative response that 'matches, fits or resonates with the child's emotional experience' (Wallin and Johnson, 2007: 106). Within this communicative, intimate interplay the infant is paid special attention to, and is recognized as a self in her own right. Such communication cues nurture 'epistemic trust' (Fonagy *et al.*, 2011), opening a channel to receive knowledge about a social and personally relevant world of culture and laying the foundations of secure attachments.

Recent research bringing together theories of communicative instinct in humans and infant observations suggests that 'preverbal human infants are prepared to receive culturally relevant knowledge from benevolent adults who are, in turn, spontaneously inclined to provide it' (Csibra and Gergely, 2011: 1149). Infants are, it seems, prepared to receive cultural knowledge that is shared through non-verbal communicative demonstrations addressed to them at a remarkably early age (Egyed *et al.*, 2013). Experiences of maltreatment, neglect or abuse, however, may result in epistemic *mis*trust and insecure attachment, linked to cognitive disadvantages and, amongst other conditions, depression (Bifulco *et al.*, 2002). As Peter Hobson (2007: 180) puts it: 'For good or ill, one's experiences of relations with others becomes a feature of one's relations with oneself.'

Such all too common experiences of early infant neglect in its many forms – of not being seen, and the repeated lived episodes of being overlooked, undervalued, spoken over, walked over, looked through – can render us with a sense of being less than solid, ethereal; and less worthy because of this. Of course this was not the experience or the case with everyone I spoke to – but difficult early years, childhoods of invisibility and descriptions of neglect and mistrust were common themes across the interviews, and are experiences all too heavily co-implicated with adult mental ill health across the length and breadth of its literature. Here is Eilish, for example, on her memory of being mothered:

> *Just [a] constant critical parent . . . she'd already broken my arm, [by that time] so that kind of sets the scene for everything that followed at the time. And she definitely didn't have a sense of me in her for example. I don't think she ever felt any connection to me at all. She didn't see me as part of her, I suggest.*

The experience of becoming mentally ill and entering into psychiatric care is also well documented, tragically, for its lack of ability to treat the whole person or to see the person behind the diagnosis – experiences which further compound the experiences of invisibility and worthlessness. Ingrid reflected on:

> *How often our problems are caused by fundamentally . . . (pause) we don't believe we are worthy of being loved or of loving . . .*

And for Aysel,

> *. . . if it wasn't for art, I think I would have gone under. It was like the colours, the shapes, the respect, the exhibitions, the acknowledgement that you are a person, that you exist, that your feelings, your thoughts are countable.*

Here is Ingrid again, talking while showing a drawing she made while in hospital:

> *There's . . . some very dark images . . . which I haven't looked at for a while which, I think I'd describe as a sense of despair, and nihilism and darkness that you can feel when you're depressed and which perhaps relates to some kind of fundamental wounding. Because although I think people easily develop unhelpful cognitive patterns when they're depressed, the depression doesn't come from nowhere I think it does come to, it does come from some kind of sense of annihilation of the self, very early on in life, some kind of deep woundedness so that was an image that describes that.*

This deep woundedness, perhaps through 'deficiencies of response' (Wright, 2009: 49) of the early environment, or through repeated experiences of being 'unseen', is, in the psychoanalytic canon, an aspect of human experience addressed through art. Wright continues:

> I suggest that artistic activity is one such way of making good the original deficit; by creating his own containing forms, the artist is saying: what I couldn't get from the other person, I am now making for myself. From this perspective, artistic activity is a means of fashioning mirroring and containing forms, and thus a way of realizing and restoring the self.

Some participants described the poignant experience of being seen through one's art with an accompanying sense of restoration of the self, and how this then released them into the daring act of disclosure. Disclosure then moved some on to the display of one's work, which, for some, like Tilly, was at first '*worse than standing in the nude*'. Disclosure and display figured as stations of the art journey with its bridging from the private, 'invisible' realm into the social domain. For many artists, this disclosure and display element of art making galvanizes; as Birdy put it, '*Once it's out there, you stand by it.*'

Disclosure and display often played an important risky but therapeutic role, with people describing these processes as simultaneously frightening *and* agentic and life-affirming, sometimes laying down a milestone in the recovery journey. In Erving Goffman's now classic touchstone work on stigma and identity, he outlines how people choose 'to display or not display' (Goffman, 1963: 42) certain personal characteristics, based on their fear of being stigmatized, and some artists experienced their habitual, even ritual concealment at last being challenged through their art practice and offered a means by which to change.

For some this was felt to be cathartic; not only a personal victory but a well overdue cocking a snook at, variously, the psychiatric monolith, the enduring merchants of stigma, or even friends and family who had been less than supportive along the way, or, as some put it, 'in denial' for their own reasons. The point of disclosure and display through one's art was often spoken of as a triumphant point – not surprisingly, considering the achievement. Both disclosure and display were invariably hard-won milestones, and the negotiation of the risk, contradictions and rewards involved in these sometimes heralded therapeutic outcomes; participants described relief, release, an enhanced sense of honesty, a feeling of being in the world and a sense of balance.

In being seen through one's art these artists may finally be achieving some sense of attunement with an other that had been felt to be missing – if not in early years experiences then almost certainly since mental ill health took hold and ushered in repeated experiences of being overlooked or wrongly seen; labelled; stigmatized; categorized; *despatched*. In disclosing through a medium of choice and delicacy, an important statement about self was being made. And in displaying, there was an important 'ta dah' moment, in which one was seen, one disclosed, and, in some cases, succeeded in making the audience comprehend, in a visceral way, '*something of the experience of being me*'. Then, moving on in a bold new way became possible:

> *Eventually the purge is over. Then you can get on and be bigger than a single label.*

> (Eilish)

An enriching expansion of relational possibilities[4]

The change that people described, from being overlooked and in some cases feeling invisible, to being seen and showing, entailed the development of trust. Some artists spoke of the importance of being able to expose one's 'ugly interior' as well as the more acceptable external façade:

> *I wanted to do a project that reflected what I'd been through so I decided to do a mask making project and in the build up to that I did these massive acrylic paintings and I actually put tights on my face and . . . you know how if you pull the tights you can disfigure your face? I put clear tights on my face and disfigured it and took pictures and then painted from those and kind of didn't tell anyone who it was and let people come round and [they were] like, 'Oh, that's so ugly', and 'That's disgusting', and then kind of just tell them it's a self-portrait and everyone was like, 'You don't look like that.' And I'd show them the photographs and say, 'Yeah, this is me. This is me, you have to believe it.' And the idea behind that was that feeling that there is something inside you that is ugly and twisted and that people don't want to look at. You know, the people don't want to know about but if they could see it they would treat you differently.*

> *Then from that I moved on to making masks and my favourite one was the rabbit of lost things; which I made out of broken and collected found objects. The idea behind that was making something beautiful out of fragments of my past and so it had nails for teeth and a broken stopwatch for an eye and massive wire ears and bits of plastic and bandages around. Often I am trying to communicate something; sometimes I will be saying, 'Help!' and sometimes I will be saying, 'Right I want you to look at this. I want you to feel uncomfortable and I want you to think why you feel uncomfortable.'*

> (Jasmine Waldorf)

In many cases trust was, and remains, a tall order, particularly where there were narrated experiences of abuse, repeated betrayal, and a history of lies and secrecy. Such betrayals and subsequent difficulties with trust are all too frequently part of the narrative of adult mental ill health. For others, mental illness had stolen upon a life in which they had enjoyed relatively stable and trustworthy relationships, and sometimes these had been collateral damage in the storm created by that illness. And for others still, their life perspective had been so altered by their experience of mental illness that old relationships and ways of relating were shed as a new identity found that these no longer fitted. Here is Charly, a young woman who has battled both alcoholism and mental ill health and has been diagnosed with Borderline Personality Disorder. She spoke ardently of her attempts to leave negative influences in her life behind her:

> *Without going too far into it, all I'll say is a lot of people showed me their true colours this year and a lot of people have let me down big time, people I thought I could trust. A lot of stuff came to light over the weekend which was my birthday when someone who I really held in high regard let the side down, and now I'm just feeling a bit confused by it all. It's made me put my back up. It's made me really quite hard and quite cold. I don't know if that's a good thing or a bad thing. It will help me get more driven and focused on the art again.*

> *But like I said, I think it's because of the BPD, I'm so sensitive to everything, and if there's negativity, even if – people don't have to say nothing, you can just pick it up – and I think where I'm living at the moment, it's not good for me. There's no life there. It's drab. I think now that's where the art's going to go. It's going to go into sort of . . . identity. It's always been there, but now I really need to revamp it . . . Here [at the art project] it's absolutely fine, because it's all these people and you're getting the vibe, but back home there's a tendency to slip into really bad habits . . .*

So amongst the narratives of people who spoke to me, often candidly, about their relationships, trusts and betrayals, there emerged a theme that will come as no surprise to anyone familiar with either mental illness or the wreckage it can leave in its episodic wake: that sometimes, as part of a recovery trajectory, one has to (re)build relationships, forge new ones, learn new ways of relating more congruent with one's (new) identity, and learn to trust even when that particular well had run dry. One further role for art making, it emerged, was as part of this process, both in terms of identity excavation and re-building and in terms of the connections with others, the social act of art making and displaying.

The process of coming to be seen by like-minded peers such as other art makers within safe spaces, disclosing to them and wider networks within gallery and community spaces and then displaying and speaking about one's work all worked as safe 'practice' grounds.

> *You just come in here and people just treat you like a human being. They don't judge you. There's never negative energy. Even if there's a few flaws, it's very like, 'well, this could be*

improved' – it's not like bang the drum blatant. It's not nasty, callous. It's not like nit-picking. And I'm not used to that. Empathy, definitely.

(Charly)

With a call to trust and be trusted within one's art group, therapeutic community, gallery space or community project, came, in some cases, the forming of attachments. For some of the participants who had a history of difficulties with relating, social functioning, trust and maintaining friendships, this opportunity, in and of itself, provided the main therapeutic impetus. For in such safe groups, nuanced 'experiments' could be made, with reciprocity, trusting and disclosing; building and repairing, at a pace which was comfortable.

As described in Chapter 3, for some, art practice itself took on a social mode, thrusting them out of their comfort zone and into new circles and ways of relating. Here is Birdy:

I started taking photographs . . . for the collages . . . and I had to go up to, like, approach (laughs) . . . members of the public . . . I had to learn how to persuade them with my manner (laughs) . . . to get them to agree to be in these scenes that I set up. Then I, I, made a short film – all about this performance with a group of drama students and street performers . . . and that was another move forward . . . because, it was hard but, it meant I, I was able to be with people for a longer period of time and build a relationship with them, daily, doing things together, interacting . . . and yeah, repairing all . . . all the cock ups I sometimes caused with my way of talking . . .

According to some attachment theorists, the 'epistemic trust' (Fonagy *et al.*, 2011) necessary for learning and creative pursuit may be achieved as a consequence of improved social relationships, and it seemed that such development of trust and attachments was another subtle by-product of art making and its engagement processes. Interestingly, attachment research also suggests that *social groups* can be regarded as attachment objects since they can offer protection and recognition to individuals (Smith *et al.*, 1999), and such group attachments rang through in people's stories. Particularly for those artists for whom attachment, intimacy, the coming to know another, being known and sustaining that relationship were ongoing fraught areas, the group seemed to offer an ideal playground (literally, a space to play with forming attachments). When the group was joined by the common purpose of art making, there was the further incentive for investment. Liz Atkin here describes the power of working with a group that is united in experiences of an illness and a creative depiction of it:

When I meet other people that are in terrible pain with it [the illness] it's very powerful to talk about the freedom that has come about through having a creative practice in this way. Maybe it provides a bit of hope to other people.

And Martha Orback:

> *Because of the interchange of ideas, because of the extra amount of bravery that I think you can have and also, yeah, I suppose it just broadens out what you are capable of.*

The artist, the group and the art making (with its products and processes) can be seen to represent a dynamic triangle. The power of this triangle can be traced again to psychoanalytic thinking; in Object Relations Theory the paternal (or third object) is seen to take up position as the one through which the merged dyadic (infant and primary caregiver) experience is challenged. Post-Kleinian theory has developed the early thinking of Freud on the Oedipal triangle in relation to thinking, and describes how the emergence of triangular space, internalized and mentally encoded (Britton, 1989; Noel-Smith, 2002), allows for dimensioned, nuanced and creative thinking – a step from the intimate merger of infant and one other, into the world. For Britton, the triangle offers the mental space to think, to imagine and tolerate a relationship between two people that exists independently of the child itself, and to think this both from within the triangle and from without. It is then possible to imagine more than one position to be known from, and from which to know others and an other. *Thirdness* signals an expansion of mental space, and as we mature, this enables more complex relating, trusting and dialectic.[5] As Froggett and colleagues (2011: 41) put it: 'The third functions as a node around which social relations and imaginative constructs are generated.' The 'aesthetic third' is thus posited, with artwork helping people to 'create an embodied, sensual connection to the world outside themselves' (2011: 92). The artwork thus provides 'a third object between themselves and others that can be shared. By animating, or re-animating, a link between individual and the cultural field, it enhances their relational capacity' (2011: 92).

This conceptualization has profound implications. For if art (or its making) functions to provide a third, through which relations can be mobilized and energized, be they relations between one's self and wider cultural experience; between the artist and other(s); between the art work and the group; or the art work and the community – then community or relational (social) art has a further role to play with regard to human wellbeing and flourishing communities. This very notion of 'flourishing' rather than 'wellbeing' is described by Mike White (2011) as being one that 'implies resilience and emergence, and it presumes inter-dependency; one cannot flourish at the expense of others'. This is a role and purpose that we may instinctively 'know' to exist, but that we are less adept at explaining. Froggett (2011: 63) also suggests that arts-based activity provides an '"aesthetic third" around which a problematic set of relationships [could] be symbolised and re-configured'.

Art making, and the other it imagines, or to which it relates in the group, thus may offer opportunities for a social mending; between one's self and others, between one and a group, and between groups and other groups, through a focus centred on the art object – and its making, or coming to be. Some artists felt this touched on what it *was* to be human. Here is Phil Baird:

Well I think it is part of being human that we do [make art], many different societies produce artworks and things that are not just purely totally functional and that it's a part of human culture and what makes us human . . . that we do make artworks of all sorts and it's a sort of soulful experience both making them and seeing other people's and so on.

People to whom I spoke also took risks for their art:

Art is . . . the primary driver . . . where art is concerned I have no shame. I would do anything to realize a piece of work. I will do all sorts of things I would never do for any other area of my life.

(Eilish)

Came to trust through its making:

I work with a group of artists and . . . erm, this has been a really big thing in terms of trust . . . I've had to . . . trust the 'encounter' . . .

(Ayden)

And found themselves involved in new relational dynamics requiring a rethinking of acceptance and respect. Mike White's (2011) observations of 'the resonance within the experience of an artwork, the aesthetic agency of participatory arts, and how arts development can harness the communal will' are echoed in Yelena's description of doing a collective painting, with which I end this chapter:

You each have a section and you start painting on your section and then you move round to the next section and you have to join each section up and you end up with one big canvas and that was incredible. It was really, really good and I liked that. That was a really great communal painting – that was joining the feeling that you were all doing the same thing and the fact that you can, despite how different you are, how different everyone's expression is. It doesn't matter what everyone's expression is because everyone has got their own expression. And you watch yourself because you have to be careful not to go over other people's lines. I want to respect that person's line. I don't want to go and put my black splodge over someone else's red dots. I want to use that for there but I want to respect it by moving it around and playing with – yeah, that was really good. That was probably one of my favourite days so far because I find I do art best when I am interacting and being with other people; that is when I do my best art.

Notes

1   Readers interested in research specific to narrative coherence in schizophrenia are referred, to, amongst others, Lysaker *et al.* (2003).
2   For further detail on a process of coming to know oneself through art readers are referred to the still highly popular and insightful classic within the art therapy canon, Marion Milner's *On Not Being Able to Paint*. First published by Heinemann in 1950, the most recent edition (2010) is published by Routledge.
3   For a useful overview of the field see Berkman *et al.* (2000).

4   L. Froggett, A. Farrier and K. Poursanidou (2011):68) 'Who cares?' Museums, Health and Wellbeing Research Project: A Study of the Renaissance North West Programme, Psychosocial Research Unit, University of Central Lancashire, 68. Available at: http://museumdevelopmentnorthwest.files.wordpress.com/2012/06/who-cares report-final-w-revisions.pdf (accessed July 2014).
5   Readers wishing to look further into Kleinian and Object Relations Theory of art are referred to Glover (2009) and Gosso (2004).

In the dark hours is about both the physical/literal and the emotional/metaphorical dark hours of my life, when I stay indoors, playing scrabble online. I only play with people I know, so it does make me feel connected to my outside world, when I can't get out and experience it with people directly.

A A	A B	A D	A E	A G	A H	A I
A L	A M	A N	A R	A S	A T	A W
A X	A Y	B A	B E	B I	B O	B Y
C H	D A	D E	D I	D O	E A	E D
E E	E F	E H	E L	E M	E N	E R
E S	E T	E X	F A	F E	F Y	G I
G O	G U	H A	H E	H I	H M	H O
I O	I F	I N	I O	I S	I T	J A
J O	K A	K I	K O	K Y	L A	L I
L O	M A	M E	M I	M M	M O	M U
M Y	N A	N E	N O	N U	N Y	O B
O D	O E	O F	O H	O I	O M	O N
O O	O P	O R	O S	O U	O W	O X
O Y	P A	P E	P I	P O	Q I	R E
S H	S I	S O	S T	T A	T E	T I
T O	U G	U H	U M	U N	U P	U R
U S	U T	W E	W O	X I	X U	Y A
Y E	Y O	Y U	Z A	Z O		

1 2 3 4 5 6 7 8 9 10 11 12 13 14 15 16 17 18 19 20 21 22 23 24 25 26 27 28

In the dark hours

7 Afterword

A singular fascination[1]

> There are many ways in which we can do better to provide true care and to build social capital and individual and social resilience. However, the arts have a special contribution to make beyond the benefits of social engagement and human kindness.
>
> (Lord Howarth of Newport, 2013)

In the silences, withdrawals and sighs of exasperation in the many conversations about art practice and mental wellbeing that were shared for this book were revealed the continuing personal and collective struggles of having a mental illness in the twenty-first century. In the pauses and raised eyebrows, the shrugs and the snorts were leaked clues about the complex nature of our interaction with art making, and the draw and pull of this singular fascination. Ethnobiologist, art theorist and self-taught scholar Ellen Dissanayake referred to the 'making special' through art, saying that:

> It may be used for anything, and anything can become an occasion for art. It may or may not be beautiful; although making special often results in 'making beautiful,' specialness also may consist of strangeness, outrageousness, or extravagance. As making special is protean and illimitable, so is art.
>
> (1995: 58)

In hearing people's stories about just how powerful this making special was, I found myself thinking over and again, how little we really understand about art making's therapeutic, restorative and identity-building powers, beyond an instinctive belief that it *has* such powers. Indeed, there is now no lack of documented projects attesting to just how powerful art can be to a person experiencing mental ill health. Documented and evaluated work from the late 1980s in the field of art engagement for psychiatric patients (Bridges and Brown, 1989; Colgan *et al.*, 1991) was amongst the first to tentatively suggest a number of possible benefits to arts engagement. One paper presented Joan to us, a 26-year-old woman with auditory hallucinations (Colgan *et al.*, 1991) whose words foretold themes which were to be found in work that followed. Her words of personal satisfaction on completing a work, boosted self-esteem, a sense of belonging and trust in the arts project and a wish to remove herself from the health professionals who 'remind her of her illness' (Colgan *et al.*, 1991: 597) may well have been spoken by any one of the people in this book. These early papers also suggest that attendance at an arts studio reduced the need to attend other psychiatric services, and thus made an early case for the possible cost-effectiveness of embedding the arts within mental health care. Attention to this particular aspect has increased in the decades since, and led to a refinement of the tools with which we measure this possible correlation (Hacking *et al.*, 2006, 2008; Spandler *et al.*, 2007; Secker *et al.*, 2009); one with clear appeal in times of straitened health provision and relentless discourse of economic 'squeeze'.

Precisely how art contributes to mental wellbeing may still be something of a mystery, yet over and above the collected stories rings a deceptively simple message: Art Works. It works on the level of personal communication and catharsis; it works to help build fragmented identities; it works to give people a routine and hands-on activity that evolves, confronts and surprises. It works to communicate; to unify parts of us and to bring us together with others; to open our eyes and show us new ways of thinking about the human condition in all its sometimes puzzling forms. There is no surprise in the message in this book that we, as a developed and compassionate society, should therefore be doing everything we can to promote art activity, broaden access to its many forms and cement an even stronger commitment to ensuring a reliable interface of art with those who need its intangible powers as part of their recovery or discovery. At the same time, we need to challenge notions that social problems can be ameliorated through therapeutic arts projects charged with enhancing 'wellbeing', a focus that reduces systemic and structural failings to individual psychology, allowing policy makers to avoid making more ambitious improvements in health and welfare. We need also to remain critical of the now catch-all term 'wellbeing' – although it is used throughout this book, I remain uneasy about the normative presumptions embedded in it, presumptions that are ageist and consumerist and which routinely overlook the multiple, layered experiences of people.

Throughout the narratives gathered for this book, themes emerge and re-emerge that largely chime with those found by a growing number of researchers in the rich field of arts and mental health. The consistency of the reported themes in such work would suggest that claims of benefits derived from arts activity have considerable validity and these benefits are not attributable to a placebo or expectation effect.

Stickley (2012: 64), for example, lists amongst other themes those of human connection; as does Parr (2006). Also documented is the role of integrating one's personal experiences and the power of having belief in the work – themes which certainly flow in and out of the stories I heard. There is also a thick strand, woven throughout the fabric of these stories, that speaks of the nuanced process of identity formation experienced through engaging with art, found too by, amongst others, Stickley *et al.* (2007) and Howells and Zelnik (2009). This identity change accompanies and triggers feelings of empowerment (Heenan, 2006) achieved through moving beyond an identity of deficit, one regarded as static, ill, medicalized. The autobiographic project involved in making art fuels and deepens this transition. Time and again I was struck by the penetrative ways in which people I interviewed spoke about their illness and their art – and while one might argue that people with a propensity to self-reflection and the metacognitive skills this may hone are *drawn to* artistic expression, it may also be that the autobiographic project that is one's art practice further enhances the self-reflection and metacognition that the making of art triggers and sustains. As to the question of whether there is a link between mental ill health and creativity, this book certainly does not claim to contribute to a case, outlined in Chapter 2, either for or against such a link. But it does reaffirm that the experience of mental ill health, in all its myriad forms and degrees, is one so unfathomable that it triggers, in its wake, a grappling to make sense of it, a search for reasons, meaning, narrative. It is also an experience whose very texture stretches the limits of the word, and may thus seek expression through other forms. One of psychiatry's most famous cases, Daniel Schreber (1842–1911) wrote in 1903 of his mental illness:

> I cannot of course count upon being fully understood because things are dealt with that cannot be expressed in human language; they exceed human understanding . . . To make myself at least somewhat comprehensible I shall have to speak much in images and similes.
>
> (2000: 16)

And this act of turning to image, to simile, to metaphor, was one described over and again in the narratives of this book. As Pippa put it, '*there's what gets left unsaid, what is left over, what I can't describe, in words . . . that's what my art deals with*'.

Part and parcel of the autobiographic project, and the reflection through which people try to make sense of and express their experience, are processes which struck me in their similarity to the processes of mentalization-based therapy. This, according to Peter Fonagy and Anthony Bateman (2007), takes as an aim that of facilitating and enhancing a psychological self-narrative. With the ability to mentalize, defined as 'the capacity to make sense of self and of others in terms of subjective states and mental processes' (Fonagy and Bateman, 2007: 83), comes an agentive sense of self, a *finding* of one's mind in contrast to losing it. Mentalization of trauma can, it is said, 'moderate the negative sequelae of psychological trauma' (Fonagy *et al.*, 1996), and the articulation of just such a moderating, healing process of coming to terms can be heard as part of the creative project spoken of in this book.

Just how our mental wellbeing; our trust and ability to maintain relationships; our sense of self and understanding of our own and others' emotional minds are interlinked with the busy interplay of neurotransmitters and hormones whose traffic is only now becoming more readily observable through technological advances in neuroscience – is the focus of the broadening and deepening research into attachment, mentalization and their evolutionary role (Fonagy *et al.*, 2011). My own personal bet for twenty-first-century breakthroughs into how we connect and how we repair through making art would be placed on the research table of what Damasio (2012) called the 'natural alliance', one that combines the tools of neuroscience with the wisdom of psychoanalytically informed understandings of the human being. I would also look there for insights into the paradox as to why, 'as Western societies have got richer, their people have become no happier' (Layard, 2011: 3). This paradox pulls in its wake questions about how we live creatively, care for one another and nurture the aptitudes that may lead to us flourishing.

Ellen Dissanayake (1995) affirmed the idea that art is for life's sake, and in her *Art and Intimacy* (2000: xiii) she boldly posits her theory of the joint origin of love and art, that singular fascination: 'The psychobiological mechanisms served by love and art . . . evolved as natural ways to satisfy essential human needs that today are frequently neglected.'

New ways of thinking about ourselves in relation to others are urgently called for, as we can no longer ignore how interconnected our health is with that of others. Professor of Public Health Phil Hanlon and colleagues (2012, 2013) put forward an urgent argument in which they are not alone, arguing that we in the developed north of the globe need to find new ways of thinking, being and doing. They remind us that hand in hand with modernity are rampant materialism, individualism, consumerism and an addiction to continuing economic growth, and that modernity's very principles and foci are harmful to health and wellbeing and inimical to social equity:

> We are separated from nature and this has led to the ecological crisis. We are separated from each other and that creates conflict and damaging forms of individualism and selfishness. We are separated from ourselves in that we tend not to be in touch with our own sense of purpose. Finally, the materialistic, objectivist conception of our world and ourselves is robbing us of a subjective connection with what might best be called 'spirit'.
>
> (Hanlon *et al.*, 2012: 238)

Our old ways of doing business with life have led to a series of crises rather than successes, and these old ways are making us and keeping us ill. It does not take an undue amount of cynicism to spot the symbiosis between capitalism in any of its various 'post' forms – and the preservation of a sick populace through the even further medicalization of society:

> The engines behind increasing medicalization are shifting from the medical profession, interprofessional or organizational contests, and social movements and interest groups to biotechnology, consumers, and managed care organizations. Doctors are still gatekeepers for medical treatment, but their role has become more subordinate in the expansion or contraction of medicalization. In short, the engines of medicalization have proliferated and are now driven more by commercial and market interests than by professional claims-makers.
>
> (Conrad, 2005: 10)

The discourse of recovery could be heard breathing throughout the narratives of this book, and, as described in Chapter 4, is one tightly interlaced with notions of empowerment and identity. This discourse feeds into the rise of positive psychology and vice versa, and a small note of caution should be added here to reiterate that in Chapter 4, where I described the double-edged nature of such a powerful discourse. Books such as this that strive to move away from a discourse of deficit and celebrate the achievements and hard-won prizes of those with disadvantaged lives can all too easily be co-opted into a broader neo-liberal tide reifying the individual and her 'personal' indomitable strength. And there is a difficult balancing act to be performed. For while it is right that we illuminate and celebrate the stories of agency and resilience in the narratives of the people who have struggled with mental illness, we also must draw attention to the ways in which creative activity is constrained or obliterated within a particular socio-political context wherein examples of those who 'go it alone' and self-help their way back into the desired 'mainstream' are used to show what can be done as the state, its welfare provision and our responsibility towards others retreat. I hope I have gone some way to presenting both pictures without reducing the stories, achievements and battles of those with whom I spoke.

Positive psychology, which began with what was an astute and timely plea that psychology re-address its focus on the deficit and pathology inherent in the human condition and shift more of its 'intellectual energy to the study of the positive aspects of human experience' (Seligman and Csikszentmihalyi, 2000), has, in the decade or more that followed, produced some valued insights. But it has also stood roundly criticized for its fuelling of a cult of positive thinking and for its 'excessively faddish enterprise' (Richardson and Guignon, 2008: 606). It has had a direct impact on the discourse of mental health and far beyond, with its persuasive and appealing messages of self-help and personal resilience arguably preventing us from seeking political and collective solutions while repackaging all social ills as personal problems. While acknowledging that 'subjective factors like determination are critical to survival and that individuals sometimes triumph over nightmarish levels of adversity' (Ehrenreich, 2010: 205), we also need to avoid what Ehrenreich, in her stinging critique of the positive thinking industry, goes on to term the 'depraved smugness' of a delusion. Through this delusion we 'ignore the role of difficult circumstances – or worse, attribute them to our own thoughts' as part of what Ahmed (2010), in another incisive critique, refers to as the 'happiness duty'.

So a further take-home message of this book is that, yes, there is an indefatigable resilience amongst many survivors of mental ill health and we have much to learn from them as we try to face the ontological insecurities and gaping voids in belief that are the very anatomy of the twenty-first century, but. That 'but' is one that pulls us back from paddling too deeply in the warm bath of the positive thinking project with its implicit, recycled Maslowian hierarchy. That well-known triangle, with creativity part of the self-actualization of its peak, still held so firmly in the sight of positive psychology, lures us into its topography while overlooking the gristle, spit and inequity that characterize its bottom two levels and the increasing difficulty of moving out of their intractable snare.

There are enduring and urgent questions that need to remain on the agenda about who and what determines mental health, who and what determines the help we get if and when we need it, and who and what determines 'quality' in one's art and mobility through the art world. The judges of normality (Foucault, 1995: 304), the policy makers of our welfare system, and the 'lovely consensus' of the art world (Perry, 2013) are a formidable array indeed. The narratives in this book hopefully help us think about the links between the laudable heights of the human endeavour and social justice; between mental health and education and social welfare; and finally, between art and social equity.

Uncertain methods and the cult of certainty

The power and impact on people's health and their lives of the making of specialness that is art remains difficult to demonstrate, let alone 'prove'. The reality and complexity of individual experience highlights what Wigram and Gold (2012) describe as a dichotomy of scientific fact and subjective experience. The effect of a phenomenon on an individual that enhances her or his sense of wellbeing may be unique to that individual – and it should not rely on our particular model of 'scientific veracity' for the effect to be accepted. We are reminded of that complexity and subjectivity by John Tusa, the former managing director of the City of London's Barbican Centre, that there are no 'cheap thrills in art . . . but there are real thrills. They come slowly, gradually, over years and as a result of effort' (Tusa, 1999: 117).

An important seminar series supported by the Economic and Social Research Council (ESRC) on Arts, Health and Wellbeing Research in 2013–2014 highlighted the need not only for continued debate about the interface of art and health, but for continued refinement of the research methodologies used in a climate where evaluation is a basic requirement of any intervention, and the pressure to build an evidence base through which to influence policy making is growing. Hacking and colleagues (2006, 2008) found, for example, that amidst a proliferation of arts activity for those with mental health difficulties, evaluation is often lacking, retrospective or inconsistent; while Kelaher and colleagues referred to the 'fear of evaluation, in that . . . it might be reductionist, and might set uncomfortable precedents in justifying art in terms of social usefulness' (2007: 2). Eades and Ager (2008) also argued that while arts projects can lead to real health gains there is a need for more consistency and rigour in evaluation if integration with mainstream health-care delivery is to be realizable. A review of studies into the role of arts in the delivery of adult social care by Consilium, in 2013, similarly found that 'although there is fairly consistent support for the role of arts in improving both physical and mental health, the considerable variation in the evaluation methodologies used to evidence impact makes it difficult to draw out conclusions'.

Part of the difficulty lies with the very nature of 'complex interventions' and the way in which art making does not readily lend itself to positivistic methods of data collection and analysis. Art making's fruits may be slow to ripen or not easily recognizable; may pop up in a field we hadn't realized had been planted; or, to really stretch the metaphor, lie dormant only to grow into something not easily traceable back to its parent seed. This book has also described how art making serves different purposes at different points of the illness and wellness trajectory; holds profoundly different meanings for different people; and is related to a person's wellbeing in minutely nuanced ways. None of this is to suggest we withdraw from the evaluating table, even if we could. But again, as noted by many, including Hacking *et al.* (2008) and Clift (2012), we need to work to refine the tools by which to evaluate and by which to interrogate that fine interface of art making and wellbeing. That said, as Mike White argues:

> The problem is not so much the lack of so called 'hard evidence', it is more a reticence until recently on behalf of the health sector and Government to see that testimonial or qualitative evidence is of significance.
>
> (cited in Devlin, 2013: 19)

There are further reasons for the limited collection of, or enthusiasm for, the kind of 'hard evidence' that is called for. The existing capacity to conduct randomized controlled trials (RCTs), the 'gold standard' of evidence-based clinical practice, is still relatively limited:

> An immediate call for more refined experimental approaches such as RCTs is premature relative to the capacity and experience of the sector and the wide range of factors that need to be accommodated for sensitive and robust evaluation.
>
> (White, 2009: 208)

A sector-wide reluctance or wariness about the risks of harnessing 'hard scientific' metrics to complex human experience is palpable, and real questions remain about just how appropriate quantitative instruments are as a means for testing the complex interrelationship between art practice and mental wellbeing. Consequently, there is a cogent call by some to revisit 'the "groundedness"' of health/illness and wellbeing in daily life' (DeNora, 2013: 5) and a case made for upholding the 'experience nearness' (Kohut, 1978; Geertz, 1974) of certain forms of 'practice near' qualitative study (Froggett and Briggs, 2012). Advocates of user-led, user-voiced research make persuasive arguments in favour of giving such qualitative evidence more credence (Faulkner and Thomas, 2002) and giving more sophisticated attention to the narrative accounts that provide 'meaning, context and perspective of the patient's predicament' (Greenhalgh and Hurwitz, 1998: 6).

But organizations involved with arts activity for the mentally ill are under increasing pressure to provide 'hard' evidence of the impact of activities and interventions to stakeholders, and of course this poses both logistical and ideological challenges. A discourse of evaluation, measurement, targets, outcomes and 'best practice' may, for example, be seen as one utilized and promoted by government as a means of exercising control. Social and political commentators have located such trends in governance in a Foucauldian framework of disciplinary govern-mentality that controls and erodes the potential political power of community-based, user-led initiatives. Evaluation, as mentioned earlier, may also be regarded as reducing the meaning of art itself to a means in which particular targets can be met, with art being seen as 'instrumental to prescribed social outcomes and public policy agendas' (Putland, 2008: 266).

In some ways, 'evidencing' the impact of arts activity on mental wellbeing is much like the proverbial nailing of jelly to a wall. It brings together the confounding difficulties of what is still felt to be a mysterious process (making art) and the still disputed and elusive qualities of what constitutes creativity, with the contested and evolving nature of our knowledge about mental wellbeing and our dissatisfaction with the instruments for measuring it – what it is; what threatens it; what ameliorates it and, to boot, the political discomfort of reductionism; instrumentalism and the pitfalls of delivering only what can be counted. What is generally agreed, however, is that 'evidence' is needed on a pragmatic level in order to press for funding for and recognition of arts activities for the mentally ill in our increasingly evidence-driven policy climate; that using a combination of qualitative and quantitative data to throw light on different aspects of the impact of art on our lives would serve research best; that complex interventions require complex and multidisciplinary thinking; and that research in this field needs to distinguish itself in its efforts to become a beacon of collaborative, participant-driven, ethically sound research with integrity. And so the task is to develop the evaluative machinery and maintain a healthy suspicion of the pressures, discourses and potential negative impacts of evaluative procedures whilst continuing to foreground the value of user-led research:

> A marriage of two types of expertise is the essential ingredient of the best mental health care: expertise by experience and expertise by profession. Psychiatrists must work in alliance with service users to find ways of integrating user-led research with EBM.
>
> (Faulkner and Thomas, 2002: 3)

This may be a tall order, but surely not one beyond the wit of the human. The current climate of busy and rich debate, participation and deliberative discourse within the arts and health 'movement' in the UK offers a positive base from which to develop a road map while remaining wary of ideas that generate more heat than light.

A third space

The people who spoke with me were deeply appreciative of the many projects, people and programmes that had helped trigger or sustain their art activity. Their message was clear, that there needs to be a funded and long-term inclusion of arts-oriented provision within mental health services and that there was no one 'modality' that trumps the others. There seemed to be no tension in the voiced need for both the provision of art therapy and other types of arts activity. Art therapy was seen as having its place – as indeed do the different *types* of art therapy. Arts activity led by practising artists, who may also have personal experience of mental ill health is valued, as is any combination of group art projects and collaborations, where both passion and compassion have secure footholds. The people with whom I spoke welcomed the students who came in to share their time and love of art; the people, some of whom were untrained volunteers, with trolleys of paints, software, cameras, buckets of colours and tubes of glue; they also welcomed opportunities for service users to go out – to colleges, universities, community venues, galleries. Sometimes, as Jake described, the simple provision of materials and a bit of private time makes a lot of difference:

> *I'd come in . . . or rather they'd bring me in . . . or I should say dragged me in (pause) and everything at that moment, it's, it's just a mess [indicates head]. I'm scared, the voices are there the lights are bright, everyone's in my face. But when . . . I ask for . . . or they bring me some pencils and paper, or whatever it might be, felt tips . . . not usually paints (laughs) that would be lovely . . . anyway, look . . . it all s l o w s down then. It dims, gets gentler. I draw.*

Best of all, when the time comes and strength and health allow, people valued the grouping, networking, sharing and making art for themselves. They advocated the maintenance and development of 'community arts provision' in its many guises, and argued that there was a need for a more equitable arts education system which had tenable and functioning connections to these. The drivers of widening participation still have work to do in ensuring a flow of diverse traffic from outside education to in – and a flow of initiatives and resources from inside education to the communities with which it shares location but sometimes little else. Narratives of the space, the place, the mode of activity and the ways in which both individuals and groups engaged with these and each other evoked Winnicott, with his enduring concept of potential space: 'the play space, the area of the transitional object and phenomena, the analytic space, the area of cultural experience, and the area of creativity' (Ogden, 1992: 203). This concept directly informs Froggett and colleagues' useful linkages to an 'aesthetic third' that we looked at in the previous chapter:

> The aesthetic third contains both something of the individual and something of the world, meaningfully conjoined. It is in the link – the experience of being meaningfully conjoined with a bit of the world that wellbeing resides.
>
> (Froggett *et al.*, 2011: 98)

The aesthetic third, concept, placemarker or aspiration, reminds us that both creativity and healing, in whatever form, require fluidity of provision, modalities that admit to uncertainty and tolerate 'emergence' (Froggett *et al.*, 2011), and environments and relationships that foster negative capability (Bion, 1970) over frenetic, perhaps meaningless certainty.

There is a tough economic case to be fought at a time of scarce funding and scared decision making. In December 2013 the BBC, using data provided under a Freedom of Information request, reported that mental health trusts in England had had their funding cut by more than 2 per cent in real terms over the previous two years, despite there being 'a genuine increase in demand' for mental health services, according to the medical director of the South London and Maudsley NHS Trust, Dr Martin Baggaley (Buchanan, 2013a, 2013b). Given such cuts in basic services, sympathy may be lost for arguments advocating arts activity, still regarded as a non-essential service. But such grim factors of a cold landscape should not prevent work being done to develop and gather 'evidence', in whatever form, in favour of the arguments for a more ideal landscape, one in which we offer a range of ways and means to each who needs or wishes it, to engage with this singular fascination and the gifts it bestows.

Note

1   'My singular fascination' was the name of an exhibition of art works at the Bethlem Gallery in 2013 by the artist Liz Atkin, one of the contributors to this book.

Whether our concern is to inhabit this world or to study it – and at root these are the same, since all inhabitants are students and all students inhabitants – our task is not to take stock of its contents but to *follow what is going on*, tracing the multiple trails of becoming, wherever they lead.

(Tim Ingold, 2011)

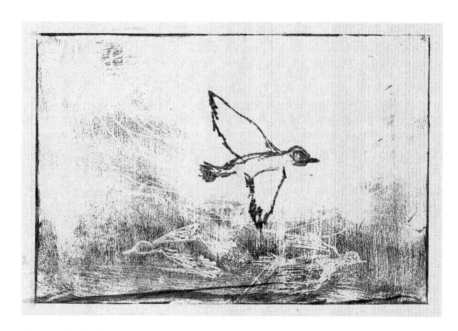

I left you in the dust

References

Ahmed, S. (2010) *The Promise of Happiness*, Durham, NC: Duke University Press

Akerman, S. and Ouellette, S.C. (2012) 'What Ricoeur's hermeneutics reveal about self and identity and aesthetic experience', *Theory and Psychology*, 22(4): 383–401

Akiskal, H.S. and Akiskal, K. (1988) 'Reassessing the prevalence of bipolar disorders: clinical significance and artistic creativity', *Psychiatry and Psychobiology*, 3: 29–36

Akiskal, K.K. and Akiskal, H.S. (2005) 'The theoretical underpinnings of affective temperaments: implications for evolutionary foundations of bipolar disorder and human nature', *Journal of Affective Disorders*, 85(1–2): 231–239

Andreasen, N.C. (1987) 'Creativity and mental illness: prevalence rates in writers and their first-degree relatives', *American Journal of Psychiatry*, 144(10): 1288–1292

Angus, J. (2002) *A Review of Evaluation in Community-Based Art for Health Activity in the UK*, London: Health Development Agency

Anthony, W.A. (1993) 'Recovery from mental illness: the guiding vision of the mental health service system in the 1990's', *Psychosocial Rehabilitation Journal*, 16(4): 11–23

Badiou, A. (2001) *Ethics*, London: Verso Books

Bakhtin, M.M. (1981) *The Dialogic Imagination*, M. Holquist (ed.), C. Emerson and M. Holquist (trans.), Austin: University of Texas Press

Baldwin, C. (2005) 'Narrative, ethics and people with severe mental illness', *Australian and New Zealand Journal of Psychiatry*, 39: 1022–1029

Banaji, S., Burn, A. and Buckingham, D. (2006) *The Rhetorics of Creativity: A Review of Literature*, London: Arts Council of England

Barron, F. and Harrington, D.M. (1981) 'Creativity, intelligence and personality', *Annual Review of Psychology*, 32: 439–476

Basch, M.F. (1981) 'Psychoanalytic interpretation and cognitive transformation', *International Journal of Psychoanalysis*, 62: 151–175

Basset, T. and Stickley, T (2010) *Voices of Experience: Narratives of Mental Health Survivors*, Chichester: Wiley-Blackwell

Bauer, J., McAdams, D.P. and Pals, J. (2008) 'Narrative identity and eudaimonic well-being', *Journal of Happiness Studies*, 9(1): 81–104

Bauman, Z. (2000) *Liquid Modernity*, Cambridge: Polity Press

BBC News, September 2013, 'Asda and Tesco withdraw Halloween patient outfit'. Available at: www.bbc.co.uk/news/uk-24278768 (accessed March 2014)

Becker G. (2001) 'The association of creativity and psychopathology: its cultural-historical origins', *Creativity Research Journal*, 13(1): 45–53

Beech, D. (2008) 'Include me out', *Art Monthly*, 315: 1–4

Beresford, P., Nettle, M. and Perring, R. (2010) 'Towards a social model of madness and distress? Exploring what service users say', Joseph Rowntree Foundation. Available at: www.jrf.org.uk/publications/social-model-madness-distress (accessed March 2014)

Berkman, L.F., Glass, T., Brissette, I. and Seeman, T.E. (2000) 'From social integration to health: Durkheim in the new millennium', *Social Science and Medicine*, 51(6): 843–857

Bersani, L. and Phillips, A. (2008) *Intimacies*, Chicago: University of Chicago Press

Bifulco, A., Moran, P.M., Ball, C. and Lillie, A. (2002) 'Adult attachment style: 2: its relationship to psychosocial depressive-vulnerability', *Social Psychiatry and Psychiatric Epidemiology*, 37: 60–67

Bion, W.R. (1962a) *Learning from Experience*, London: Heinemann; New York: Basic Books

Bion, W.R. (1962b) 'A theory of thinking', in E. Bott Spillius (ed.) *Melanie Klein Today: Developments in Theory and Practice, Volume 1: Mainly Theory*, London: Routledge, 1988

Bion, W.R. (1970) *Attention and Interpretation*, London: Karnac Books

Bishop, C. (2006) *The Social Turn: Collaboration and Its Discontents, Art Forum*, 2006: 178–183

Bishop, C. (2012) *Artificial Hells: Participatory Art and the Politics of Spectatorship*, London: Verso Books

Bollas, C. (1987) *The Shadow of the Object: Psychoanalysis of the Unthought Known*, New York: Columbia University Press

Bonney, S. and Stickley, T. (2008) 'Recovery and mental health: a review of the British literature', *Journal of Psychiatric and Mental Health Nursing*, 15: 140–153

Bourdieu, P. (1977) *Outline of a Theory of Practice*, New York: Cambridge University Press

Bourdieu, P. (1993) *The Field of Cultural Production*, Cambridge: Polity Press

Breuer, J. and Freud, S. (1955) 'Studies on hysteria', in *The Complete Psychological Works of Sigmund Freud*, J. Strachey (ed. and trans.), Standard Edition, Volume 2, London: Hogarth Press

Bridges, K. and Brown, L. (1989) 'Psychiatric patients work alongside artists on prize-winning project', *British Medical Journal*, 299: 532

Britton, R. (1989) 'The missing link: parental sexuality in the Oedipus Complex', in J. Steiner (ed.) *The Oedipus Complex Today*, London: Karnac Books

Broderick, S. (2011) 'Arts practices in unreasonable doubt? Reflections on understandings of arts practices in healthcare contexts', *Arts & Health*, 3(2): 95–109

Brown, L. (2012) 'Is art therapy?' in T. Stickley (ed.) *Qualitative Research in Arts and Mental Health*, Ross-on-Wye: PCCS Books, 2: 22–41

Bruner, J. [1986] (2005) *Actual Minds, Possible Worlds*, Cambridge, MA: Harvard University Press

Buchannan, M. (2013a) 'Funds cut for mental health trusts in England', BBC News. Available at: www.bbc.co.uk/news/health-25331644 (accessed March 2014)

Buchannan, M. (2013b) 'England's mental health services "in crisis"', BBC News. Available at: www.bbc.co.uk/news/health-24537304 (accessed March 2014)

Burch, G.St.J., Pavelis, C., Hemsley, D.R. and Corr, P.J. (2006) 'Schizotypy and creativity in visual artists', *British Journal of Psychology*, 97: 177–190

Bury, M.R. (1982) 'Chronic illness as biographical disruption', *Sociology of Health and Illness*, 4(2): 167–182

Bury, M.R. (1991) 'The sociology of chronic illness: a review of research and prospects', *Sociology of Health and Illness*, 13(4): 451–468

Bury, M.R. (2001) 'Illness narratives: fact or fiction?' *Society of Health and Illness*, 23(3): 263–285

Butler, J. (2005) *Giving an Account of Oneself*, New York: Fordham University Press

Camic, P.M. (2008) 'Playing in the mud: health psychology, the arts and creative approaches to health care', *Journal of Health Psychology*, 13: 287–298

Charmaz, K. (2002) 'Stories and silences: disclosures and self in chronic illness', *Qualitative Inquiry*, 8(3): 302–328

Claridge, G.A. (1993) 'When is psychoticism psychoticism? And how does it really relate to creativity?' *Psychological Inquiry*, 4(3): 184–188

Claridge, G.A. (1998) 'Creativity and madness: clues from modern psychiatric diagnosis', in A. Steptoe (ed.) *Genius and the Mind: Studies of Creativity and Temperament*, Oxford: Oxford University Press, 10: 227–250

Clift, S. (2012) 'Creative arts as a public health resource: moving from practice-based research to evidence-based practice', *Perspectives in Public Health*, 132: 120–127.

Cohen, B.M. (1990) 'Diagnostic drawing series', in I. Jakab (ed.) *Stress Management through Art: Proceedings of the International Congress of Psychopathology of Expression*, Boston: American Society for the Psychopathology of Expression, 123–130

Colgan, S., Bridges, K., Brown, L. and Faragher, B. (1991) 'A tentative start: evaluation of alternative forms of care for chronic users of psychiatric services', *Psychiatric Bulletin*, 15: 596–598

Comte, A. (1853) *The Positive Philosophy of Auguste Comte, Volume 1*, H. Martineau (trans.), Michigan: University of Michigan, Appleton & Company

Conrad, P. (2005) 'The shifting engines of medicalization', *Journal of Health and Social Behaviour*, 46(1): 3–14

Consilium (2013) 'What do we know about the role of arts in the delivery of social care?' Published by Skills for Care. Available at: www.skillsforcare.org.uk/Document-library/ NMDS-SC,-workforce-intelligence-and-innovation/Research/Arts-and-social-care/ Briefing-Paper-FINAL-010713.pdf (accessed March 2014)

Couser, G.T. (1997) *Recovering Bodies: Illness, Disability, and Life Writing*, Madison, WI: University of Wisconsin Press

Cropley, A.J. (2010) 'The dark side of creativity: what is it?' in D.H. Cropley, A.J. Cropley, J.C. Kaufman and M.A. Runco (eds) *The Dark Side of Creativity*, Cambridge, MA: Cambridge University Press, 1: 1–14

Crossley, M.L. (2000) 'Narrative psychology, trauma and the study of self/identity', *Theory and Psychology*, 10(4): 527–546

Csibra, G. and Gergely, G. (2011) 'Natural pedagogy as evolutionary adaptation', *Philosophical Transactions of the Royal Society*, 366(1567): 1149–1157

Csikszentmihalyi, M. (1993) 'Does overinclusiveness equal creativity?' *Psychological Inquiry*, 4(3): 188–189

Csikszentmihalyi, M. (1997) *Creativity: Flow and the Psychology of Discovery and Invention*, New York: HarperCollins

Csikszentmihalyi, M. and Csikszentmihalyi, I.S. (eds) (1988) *Optimal Experience: Psychological Studies of Flow in Consciousness*, Cambridge, MA: Cambridge University Press

Csordas, T.J. (2012) 'Psychoanalysis and phenomenology', *Ethos*, 40(1): 54–74.

Dahlberg, K., Dahlberg, H. and Nystrom, M. (2008) *Reflective Lifeworld Research*, 2nd edn, Lund, Sweden: Studentliteratur

Dalgleish, T., Navrady, L., Bird, E., Hill, E., Dunn, B.D. and Golden, A. (2013) 'Method-of-loci as a mnemonic device to facilitate access to self-affirming personal memories for individuals with depression', *Clinical Psychological Science*, 1(2): 156–162

Damasio, A. (2012) 'Neuroscience and psychoanalysis: a natural alliance', in E. Laufer, Guest Editor, Special Issue: *On the Frontiers of Psychoanalysis and Neuroscience: Essays in Honor of Eric R. Kandel, The Psychoanalytic Review*, 99(4): 591–595

Davidson, L., Rakfeldt, J. and Strauss, J. (2010) *The Roots of the Recovery Movement in Psychiatry: Lessons Learned*, Chichester: Wiley-Blackwell

Daykin, N. and Byrne, E. (2006) 'The impact of visual arts and design on the health and wellbeing of patients and staff in mental healthcare: a systematic review of the literature'. Available at: http://hsc.uwe.ac.uk/net/research/Data/Sites/1/GalleryImages/Research/Final%20report%20on%20the%20literature%20review.pdf (accessed March 2014)

Deleuze, G., Guattari, F. and Massumi, B. (2011) *A Thousand Plateaus*, London: Continuum International

DeNora, T. (2013) '"Time after time", A Quali-T method for assessing music's impact on well-being', *International Journal of Qualitative Studies in Health and Wellbeing*, 1: 1–13

Derrida, J. (2005) *Writing and Difference*, A. Bass (trans.), London: Routledge

Devlin, P. (2013) 'Restoring the balance: the effect of arts participation on wellbeing and health', Voluntary Arts England. Available at: www.voluntaryarts.org/wp-content/uploads/2011/10/Restoring-the-Balance.pdf (accessed March 2014)

Dewey, J. [1934] (2009) *Art as Experience*, New York: Perigee Books

Dillon, J. and May, R. (2003) *Reclaiming Experience, Openmind*, March/April, 119–120

Dissanayake, E. (1995) *Homo Aestheticus: Where Art Comes from and Why*, Seattle: University of Washington Press

Dissanayake, E. (2000) *Art and Intimacy: How the Arts Began*, Seattle: University of Washington Press

Drake, J.E. and Winner, E. (2012) 'Confronting sadness through art-making: distraction is more beneficial than venting', *Psychology of Aesthetics, Creativity, and the Arts*, 6(3): 255–261

Dunne, J. (1995) 'Beyond sovereignty and deconstruction: the storied self', *Philosophy and Social Criticism*, 21: 137–157

Eades, G. and Ager, J. (2008) 'Time being: difficulties in integrating arts in health', *Journal of the Royal Society for the Promotion of Health*, 128(2): 62–67

Eames, P. (2003) *Creative Solutions and Social Inclusion: Culture and the Community*, Wellington: Steele Roberts Ltd

Edwards, D. (2004) *Art Therapy*, London: Sage Publications

Egyed, K., Király, I. and Gergely, G. (2013) 'Communicating shared knowledge', *Infancy, Psychological Science*, 24: 1348–1353

Ehrenreich, B. (2010) *Smile or Die: How Positive Thinking Fooled America and the World*, London: Granta Books

Ehrenzweig, A. (1971) *The Hidden Order of Art*, Los Angeles: University of California Press

Eigen, M. (2005) *Emotional Storm*, Middletown, CT: Wesleyan University Press

Ellenberger, H.F. (1994) *The Discovery of the Unconscious*, London: Fontana

Eysenck, H.J. (1996) 'The measurement of creativity', in M.A. Boden (ed.) *Dimensions of Creativity*, Cambridge, MA: MIT Press, 199–242

Eysenck, H.J. and Eysenck S.B.G. (1978) 'Psychopathy, personality and genetics', in R.D. Hare and D. Schalling (eds) *Psychopathic Behaviour: Approaches to Research*, London: Wiley, 197–223

Faulkner, A. (2004) *The Ethics of Survivor Research: Guidelines for the Ethical Conduct of Research Carried out by Mental Health Service Users and Survivors*, Bristol: The Policy Press

Faulkner, A. and Thomas, P. (2002) 'User led research and evidence-based medicine', *British Journal of Psychiatry*, 180: 1–3

Finlay, L. (2014) 'Engaging phenomenological analysis', *Qualitative Research in Psychology*, 11(2): 121–141

Flaherty, A. (2007) 'Frontotemporal and dopaminergic control of idea generation and creative drive', *Journal of Comparative Neurology*, 493(1): 147–153

Folley, B.S. and Park, S. (2005) 'Verbal creativity and schizotypal personality in relation to prefrontal hemispheric laterality; a behavioural and near-infrared optical imaging (NIROT) study', *Schizophrenia Research*, 80(2–3): 271–282

Fonagy, P. and Bateman, A.W. (2007) 'Mentalizing and borderline personality disorder', *Journal of Mental Health*, 16(1): 83–101

Fonagy, P., Leigh, T., Steele, M., Steele, H., Kennedy, R., Mattoon, G., *et al.* (1996) 'The relation of attachment status, psychiatric classification and response to psychotherapy', *Journal of Consulting and Clinical Psychology*, 64: 22–31

Fonagy, P., Gergely, G. and Target, M. (2007) 'The parent–infant dyad and the construction of the subjective self', *Journal of Child Psychology and Psychiatry*, 48(3/4): 288–328

Fonagy, P., Bateman, A. and Bateman, A. (2011) 'The widening scope of mentalizing: a discussion', *Psychology and Psychotherapy: Theory, Research and Practice*, 84(1): 98–110

Foucault, M. (1967) *Madness and Civilization*, London: Routledge

Foucault, M. (1995) *Discipline and Punish: The Birth of the Prison*, 2nd edn, A. Sheridan (trans.), London: Vintage Books

Foucault, M. (2009) *A History of Madness*, London: Routledge

Frank, A.W. (1995) *The Wounded Storyteller*, Chicago: University of Chicago Press

Freud, S. (1910) *Leonardo da Vinci and a Memory of His Childhood, The Complete Psychological Works of Sigmund Freud*, J. Strachey (ed. and trans.), Standard Edition, Volume 11, London: Hogarth Press, 59–137

Freud, S. (1914a) *The Moses of Michelangelo, The Complete Psychological Works of Sigmund Freud*, J. Strachey (ed. and trans.), Standard Edition, Volume 13, London: Hogarth Press, 211–238

Freud, S. (1914b) 'Remembering, repeating and working-through (further recommendations on the technique of psycho-analysis II)', in *The Complete Psychological Works of Sigmund Freud*, J. Strachey (ed. and trans.), Standard Edition, Volume 12 (1911–1913), London: Hogarth Press

Freud, S. (1927) *Dostoevsky and Parricide, The Complete Psychological Works of Sigmund Freud*, J. Strachey (ed. and trans.), Standard Edition, Volume 21, London: Hogarth Press, 177–196

Freud, S. [1908] (1973) 'Creative writers and day-dreaming', in *The Complete Psychological Works of Sigmund Freud*, J. Strachey (ed. and trans.), Standard Edition, Volume 9, London: Hogarth Press, 143

Freyd, J.J., Klest, B. and Allard, C.B. (2005) 'Betrayal trauma: relationship to physical health, psychological distress and a written disclosure intervention', *Journal of Trauma & Dissociation*, 6(3): 83–104

Frie, R. (2011) 'Identity, narrative, and lived experience after postmodernity: between multiplicity and continuity', *Journal of Phenomenological Psychology*, 42(1): 46–60

Froggett, L. (2011) 'Artistic output as intersubjective third', in S. Clarke, H. Hahn and P. Hoggett (eds) *Object Relations and Social Relations: The Implications of the Relational Turn in Psychoanalysis*, London: Karnac Books, 5: 87–107

Froggett, L. and Briggs, S. (2012) 'Practice-near and practice-distant methods in human services research', *Journal of Research Practice*, 8(2), 1–17

Froggett, L. and Hollway, W. (2010) 'Psychosocial research analysis and scenic understanding', *Psychoanalysis, Culture & Society*, 15(3): 281–301

Froggett, L., Little, R., Roy, A. and Witaker, L. (2011) 'New model visual arts organisations and social engagement', Psychosocial Research Unit, University of Central Lancashire. Available at: www.artsandhealth.ie/wp-content/uploads/2013/02/New-Model-Visual-Arts-Organisations-and-Social-Engagement.pdf (accessed March 2014)

Fromm, E. (2002) *The Sane Society*, London: Routledge

Frosh, S. (2002) *After Words: The Personal in Gender, Culture and Psychotherapy*, Basingstoke: Palgrave Macmillan

Furnham, A., Batey, M., Anand, K. and Manfield, J. (2008) 'Personality, hypomania, intelligence and creativity', *Personality and Individual Differences*, 44: 115–121

Gabora, L. and Holmes, N. (2010) 'Dangling from a tassel on the fabric of socially constructed reality: reflections on the creative writing process', in D.H. Cropley, A.J. Cropley, J.C. Kaufman and M.A. Runco (eds) *The Dark Side of Creativity*, Cambridge, MA: Cambridge University Press, 15: 227–296

Geddes, J. (2004) 'Art and mental health: building the evidence base', in J. Cowling (ed.) *For Art's Sake. Society and the Arts in the 21st Century*, London: IPPR, 64–74

Geertz, C. (1974) 'From the native's point of view: on the nature of anthropological understanding', *Bulletin of the American Academy of Arts and Sciences*, 28(1): 26–45

Gergen, K.J. (1990) 'Therapeutic professions and the diffusion of deficit', *Journal of Mind and Behaviour*, 11: 353–368

Gerhardt, S. (2010) *The Selfish Society: How We All Forgot to Love One Another and Made Money Instead*, London: Simon & Schuster

Ghadirian, A.M., Gregoire, P. and Kosmidis, H. (2001) 'Creativity and the evolution of psychopathologies', *Creativity Research Journal*, 13(2): 145–214

Gladding, S.T. and Newsome, D.W. (2003) 'Art in counseling', in C.A. Malchiodi (ed.), *Handbook of Art Therapy*, New York: Guilford Press, 243–253

Glaveanu, V. (2010) 'Principles for a cultural psychology of creativity', *Culture & Psychology*, 16: 147–163

Glazer, E. (2009) 'Rephrasing the madness and creativity debate: what is the nature of the creative construct?' *Personality and Individual Differences*, 46: 755–764

Glicksohn, J., Alon, A., Perlmutter, A. and Purisman, R. (2001) 'Symbolic and syncretic cognition among schizophrenics and visual artists', *Creativity Research Journal*, 13(2): 133–143

Glover, N. (2009) *Psychoanalytic Aesthetics: An Introduction to the British School*, London: Harris Meltzer Trust and Karnac Books

Goffman, E. (1963) *Stigma: Notes on the Management of Spoiled Identities*, New York: Simon & Schuster.

Good, B.J. (2012) 'Phenomenology, psychoanalysis, and subjectivity in Java', *Ethos*, 40(1): 24–36

Goodwin, F.K. and Jamison, K.R. (eds) (2007) *Manic-Depressive Illness: Bipolar Disorders and Recurrent Depression*, 2nd edn, New York: Oxford University Press

Gosso, S. (ed.) (2004) *Psychoanalysis and Art: Kleinian Perspectives*, London: Karnac Books

Greene, M. (1995) *Releasing the Imagination: Essays on Education, the Arts and Social Change*, San Francisco: Jossey-Bass

Greenhalgh, T. and Hurwitz, B. (eds) (1998) *Narrative Based Medicine: Dialogue and Discourse in Clinical Practice*, London: BMJ Books

Grossmann, T., Oberecker, R., Koch, S.P. and Friederici, A.D. (2010) 'The developmental origins of voice processing in the human brain', *Neuron*, 65(6): 852–858

Guarneri, M. (2007) *The Heart Speaks: A Cardiologist Reveals the Secret Language of Healing*, New York: Simon & Schuster

Guilfoyle, M. (2005) 'From therapeutic power to resistance? Therapy and cultural hegemony', *Theory and Psychology*, 15(1): 101–124

Gwinner, K., Knox, M. and Hacking, S. (2010) 'The place for a contemporary artist with a mental illness', *Journal of Public Mental Health*, 8(4): 29–37

Habermas, J. (1984) *Theory of Communicative Action, Volume One: Reason and the Rationalization of Society*, Thomas A. McCarthy (trans.), Boston, MA: Beacon Press

Hacking, I. (2013) 'Lost in the forest', *London Review of Books*, 35(15) (8 August)

Hacking, S. and Foreman, D. (2001) 'Psychopathology in paintings: a meta-analysis of studies using paintings by psychiatric patients', *British Journal of Medical Psychology*, 74: 35–45

Hacking, S., Foreman, D. and Belcher, J. (1996) 'The descriptive assessment for psychiatric art, a new way of quantifying paintings by psychiatric patients', *Journal of Nervous and Mental Disease*, 184(7): 425–430

Hacking, S., Secker, J., Kent, L., Shenton, J. and Spandler, H. (2006) 'Mental health and arts participation: the state of art in England', *Journal of the Royal Society of Health Promotion*, 126(3): 121–127

Hacking, S., Secker, J., Spandler, H., Kent, L. and Shenton, J. (2008) 'Evaluating the impact of participatory art projects for people with mental health needs', *Health and Social Care in the Community*, 16(6): 638–648

Hanlon, P., Carlisle, S., Hannah, M., Lyon, A. and Reilly, D. (2012) 'A perspective on the future public health practitioner', *Perspectives in Public Health 2012*, 132(5): 235–239

Hanlon, P., Carlisle, S., Hannah, M., Lyon, A. and Reilly, D. (2013) 'A perspective on the future public health: an integrative and ecological framework', *Perspectives in Public Health 2012*, 132(6): 313–319

Harper, D. (2002) 'The tyranny of expert language', *Open Mind*, 113: 8–9

Harper, D. and Speed, E. (2012) 'Uncovering recovery: the resistible rise of recovery and resilience', *Studies in Social Justice*, 6(1): 9–25

Hartill, G. (1998) 'The web of words: collaborative writing and mental health', in C. Hunt and F. Sampson (eds) *The Self on the Page: Theory and Practice of Creative Writing in Personal Development*, London: Jessica Kingsley

Healy, D. (2008) *Mania: A Short History of Bipolar Disorder*, Baltimore, MD: Johns Hopkins University Press

Hebron, D. and Taylor, K. (2012) 'A new age: the changing face of health funding for arts activity, with, by and for older people in England', London Arts and Health Forum, commissioned by the Baring Foundation

Heenan, D. (2006) 'Art as therapy: an effective way of promoting positive mental health?' *Disability & Society*, 21(2): 179–191

Hegel, G.W.F. [1835] (1975) *Hegel's Aesthetics, Lectures on Fine Art: Volume 1*, T.M. Knox (trans.), Oxford: Oxford University Press

Heisenberg, W. (1971) *Physics and Beyond, Encounters and Conversations*, New York: Harper & Row

Hennessey, B.A. and Amabile, T.M. (2010) 'Creativity', *Annual Review of Psychology*, 61: 569–598

Henriques, J., Hollway, W., Urwin, C., Venn, C. and Walkerdine, V. (1998) *Changing the Subject: Psychology, Social Regulation and Subjectivity*, London: Routledge

Hill, A. (1945) *Art Versus Illness: A Story of Art Therapy*, London: Allen & Unwin

Hinshaw, S. (2011) *The Mark of Shame: Stigma of Mental Illness and an Agenda for Change*, New York: Oxford University Press

Hobson, P. (2007) *The Cradle of Thought: Exploring the Origins of Thinking*, London: Pan Macmillan

Hogan, S. (2001) *Healing Arts: The History of Art Therapy*, London: Jessica Kingsley

Hollway, W. and Jefferson, T. (2000) *Doing Qualitative Research Differently: Free Association, Narrative and the Interview Method*, London: Sage Publications

Holly, M.A. (2013) *The Melancholy Art*, Princeton, NJ: Princeton University Press

Holmes, J. (2014) 'Countertransference in qualitative research: a critical appraisal', *Qualitative Research*, 14(2): 166–183

Hornstein, G. (2009) *Agnes's Jacket: A Psychologist's Search for the Meanings of Madness*, New York: Rodale Books

Howells, V. and Zelnik, T. (2009) 'Making art: a qualitative study of personal and group transformation in a community arts studio', *Psychiatric Rehabilitation Journal*, 32(3): 215–222

Ingold, T. (2011) *Being Alive: Essays on Movement, Knowledge and Description*, London: Routledge

Jacques, E. (1965) 'Death and the mid-life crisis', in E.B. Spillus (ed.) (1990) *Melanie Klein Today, Volume 2: Mainly Practice*, London: Routledge

Jamison, K.R. (1989) 'Mood disorders and patterns of creativity in British writers and artists', *Psychiatry*, 52: 125–134

Kalian, M., Lerner, V. and Witztum, E. (2002) 'Creativity an affective illness, letter to the editor', *American Journal of Psychiatry*, 159(4): 675–676

Karlsson, J.L. (1970) 'Genetic association of giftedness and creativity with schizophrenia', *Hereditas*, 66: 177–182

Kelaher, M., Berman, N., Joubert, L., Curry, S., Jones, R., Stanley, J. and Johnson, V. (2007) 'Methodological approaches to evaluating the impact of community arts on health', *UNESCO Observatory E-Journal*, 1: 1–18

Kelaher, M., Dunt, D., Brman, N., Curry, S., Joubert, L. and Johnson, V. (2013) Evaluating the health impacts of participation in Australian community arts groups', *Health Promotion International*, 30 January 2013: Epub ahead of print (accessed March 2014)

Kester, G. (1995) 'Aesthetic evangelists: conversion and empowerment in contemporary community art', *Afterimage*, 22: 5–11

Kester, G. (1997) 'Aesthetics after the end of art: an interview with Susan Buck-Morss (Aesthetics and the Body Politic)', *Art Journal*, 56(1): 38–45

Kester, G. (2004) *Conversation Pieces: Community and Communication in Modern Art*, Berkeley, CA: University of California Press

Kester, G. (2012) 'The game is up: programmers, patronage and the neo-liberal state', Introduction to *Gallery as Community: Art, Education, Politics*, Whitechapel Gallery, London: 2012. Available at: www.grantkester.net/resources/Whitechapel+Introduction.pdf (accessed July 2014)

Killick, K. (1995) 'Working with psychotic processes in art therapy', in J. Ellwood (ed.) *Psychosis: Understanding and Treatment*, London: Jessica Kingsley, 8: 105–119

Kinney, D.K., Richards, R., Lowing, P.A., Leblanc, D., Zimbalist, M.E. and Harlan, P. (2001) 'Creativity in offspring of schizophrenic and control parents: an adoption study', *Creativity Research Journal*, 13(1): 17–25

Klein, M. (1946) 'Notes on some schizoid mechanisms', *International Journal of Psychoanalysis*, 27: 99–110, reprinted in *Envy and Gratitude and Other Works 1946–1963*, London: Virago, 1988, 1–24

Klein, M. (1958) 'On the development of mental functioning', in *Envy and Gratitude and Other Works*, London: Hogarth Press, 1975, 236–246

Kleinman, A. (1988) *The Illness Narratives: Suffering, Healing, and the Human Condition*, New York: Basic Books

Kleinman, A. and Good, B. (eds) (1992) *Culture and Depression: Studies on the Anthropology and Cross-Cultural Psychiatry of Affect and Disorder*, Berkeley, CA: University of California Press

Koh, C. (2006) 'Reviewing the link between creativity and madness: a postmodern perspective', *Educational Research and Reviews*, 1(7): 213–221

Kohut, H. (1978) 'The psychoanalyst in the community of scholars', in P.H. Ornstein (ed.) *The Search for the Self: Selected Writings of Heinz Kohut: 1950–1978*, New York: International Universities Press, 2: 685–724

Kristeva, J. (1989) *Black Sun: Depression and Melancholia*, L. Roudiez (trans.), New York: Columbia University Press

Kwon, M. (2002) *One Place after Another: Site Specific Art and Locational Identity*, Cambridge, MA: MIT Press

Kyaga, S., Landén, M., Boman, M., Hultman, C.M., Långström, N. and Lichtenstein, P. (2013) 'Mental illness, suicide and creativity: 40-year prospective total population study', *Journal of Psychiatric Research*, 47(1): 83–90

Lane, R.E. (2000) *The Loss of Happiness in Market Economies*, New Haven and London: Yale University Press.

Langdridge, D. (2007) *Phenomenological Psychology: Theory, Research and Method*, Harlow, Essex: Pearson

Langer, S.K. (1930) *The Practice of Philosophy*, New York: Henry Holt

Langer, S.K. (1957) *Problems of Art*, New York: Scribner

Layard, R. (2011) *Happiness: Lessons from a New Science*, 2nd edn, London: Penguin

Lombroso, C. (1891) *The Man of Genius*, London: Walter Scott Publishing Ltd

López de la Torre, A.L. (2013) E-mail interview, 21 April 2013

Love, K. (2005) 'The experience of art as a living through of language', in G. Butt (ed.) *After Criticism: New Responses to Art and Performance*, Oxford: Blackwell Publishing, 156–176

Ludwig, A.M. (1995) *The Price of Greatness: Resolving the Creativity and Madness Controversy*, New York: Guilford Press

Lysaker, P., Lancaster R. and Lysaker, J. (2003) 'Narrative transformation as an outcome in the psychotherapy of schizophrenia', *Psychology and Psychotherapy: Theory, Research and Practice*, 76(3): 285–299

MacCallum, E.J. (2002) 'Othering and psychiatric nursing', *Journal of Psychiatric and Mental Health Nursing*, 9: 87–94

Mahler, M. (1968) *On Human Symbiosis and the Vicissitudes of Individuation*, New York: International Universities Press

Marmot, M. and Wilkinson, R. (eds) (2005) *Social Determinants of Health*, Oxford: Oxford University Press

Martin, L.L., Ward, D.W., Achee, J.W. and Wyer, R.S. (1993) 'Mood as input: people have to interpret the motivational implications of their moods', *Journal of Personality and Social Psychology*, 64(3): 317–326.

Matarasso, F. (1997) *Use or Ornament? The Social Impact of Participation in the Arts*, Stroud, Glos.: Comedia

Matarasso, F. (2013) 'Creative progression: reflections on quality in participatory arts', *UNESCO Observatory, Multi-Disciplinary Journal in the Arts*, 3(3): 1–15. Available at: http://web.education.unimelb.edu.au/UNESCO/ejournal/ejournal_vol3iss3.html (accessed March 2014)

McAdams, D.P. (2008) 'Personal narratives and the life story', in O.P. John, R.W. Robins and L.A. Pervin (eds) *Handbook of Personality: Theory and Research*, 3rd edn, New York: Guilford, 8: 242–262

McAdams, D.P., Reynolds, J., Lewis, M., Patten, A.H. and Bowman, P.J. (2001) 'When bad things turn good and good things turn bad: sequences of redemption and contamination in life narrative and their relation to psychosocial adaptation in midlife adults and in students', *Personality and Social Psychology Bulletin*, 27(4): 474–485

McCrory, E., De Brito, S. and Viding, E. (2012) 'The link between child abuse and psychopathology: a review of neurobiological and genetic research', *Journal of the Royal Society of Medicine*, 105(4): 151–156

McCulloch, A. (2012) *Creativity and Mental Illness – An Exercise in Clarification*, Mental Health Foundation. Available at: www.mentalhealth.org.uk/our-news/blog/121030creativity/ (accessed March 2014)

McKenzie, K. and Harpham, T. (eds) (2006) *Social Capital and Mental Health*, London: Jessica Kingsley

Merli, P. (2002) 'Evaluating the social impact of participation in arts activities. A critical review of Francois Matarasso's "Use or Ornament?"' *International Journal of Cultural Policy*, 8(1): 107–118

Miller, G.F. and Tal, I.R. (2007) 'Schizotypy versus openness and intelligence as predictors of creativity', *Schizophrenia Research*, 93: 317–324

Millon, T. (2004) *Masters of the Mind: Exploring the Story of Mental Illness from Ancient Times to the New Millennium*, New York: John Wiley & Sons

Milner, M. (1950) *On Not Being Able to Paint*, 2nd edn, London: Heinemann

Morgan, A. and Swann, C. (eds) (2004) 'Social capital for health: issues of definition, measurement and links to health', Health Development Agency. Available from: www.nice.org.uk/ (accessed March 2014)

Mula, M. and Trimble, M.R. (2009) 'Music and madness: neuropsychiatric aspects of music', *Clinical Medicine, Journal of the Royal College of Physicians*, 9(1): 83–86

Murphy, C. (2009) 'The link between artistic creativity and psychopathology: Salvador Dali', *Personality and Individual Differences*, 46(8): 765–774

Neelands, J. and Boyun, C. (2010) 'The English model of creativity: cultural politics of an idea', *International Journal of Cultural Policy*, 16(3): 287–304

Nelson, B. and Rawlings, D. (2010) 'Relating schizotypy and personality to the phenomenology of creativity', *Schizophrenia Bulletin*, 36(2): 388–399

Nettle, D. (2001) *Strong Imagination: Madness, Creativity and Human Nature*, Oxford: Oxford University Press

Nettle, D. (2006) 'Schizotypy and mental health amongst poets, visual artists and mathematicians', *Journal of Research in Personality*, 40: 876–890

Nisbet, J.F. (1900) *The Insanity of Genius and the General Inequality of Human Faculty: Physiologically Considered*, 4th edn, London: Grant Richards

Noel-Smith, K. (2002) 'Time and space as "necessary forms of thought"', *Free Associations*, 9(51): 394–442

Ogden, T.H. (1992) *The Matrix of the Mind: Object Relations and the Psychoanalytic Dialogue*, London: Karnac Books

Oliver, M. and Barnes, C. (2012) *The New Politics of Disablement*, London: Palgrave Macmillan

Pajaczkowska, C. (2007) 'On humming: reflections on Marion Milner's contribution to psychoanalysis', in L. Caldwell (ed.) *Winnicott and the Psychoanalytic Tradition*, London: Karnac Books, 3: 33–48

Park, M. (2010) *Art in Madness, Dr W.A.F. Browne's Collection of Patient Art at Crichton Royal Institution, Dumfries*, Dumfries: Dumfries and Galloway Health Board

Parker, I. (2010) 'The place of transference in psychosocial research', *Journal of Theoretical and Philosophical Psychology*, 30(1): 17–31

Parker, R. and Pollock, G. (1981) *Old Mistresses: Women, Art and Ideology*, London: Routledge & Kegan Paul

Parr, H. (2006) 'Mental health, the arts and belongings', *Transactions of the Institute of British Geographers*, 31(2): 150–166

Parr, H. (2012) 'The arts and mental health: creativity and inclusion', in T. Stickley (ed.) *Qualitative Research in Arts and Mental Health*, Ross-on-Wye: PCCS Books

Passeron, J.C. and Bourdieu, P. (1990) *Reproduction in Education, Society and Culture*, London: Sage

Perkins, R. and Slade, M. (2012) 'Recovery in England: transforming statutory services?' *International Review of Psychiatry*, 24(1): 29–39

Perry, G. (2013) *Playing to the Gallery – Democracy Has Bad Taste*, BBC Radio 4, Reith Lectures 1

Pies, R. (2007) 'The historical roots of the "bipolar spectrum": did Aristotle anticipate Kraepelin's broad concept of manic depression?' *Journal of Affective Disorders*, 100: 7–11

Poincaré, H. (1910) 'The future of mathematics', *The Monist*, 20(1): 76–92. Available at: www.jstor.org/stable/27900234 (accessed March 2014)

Polkinghorne, D. (1988) *Narrative Knowing and the Human Sciences*, Albany, NY: State University of New York Press

Porter, R. (2002) *Madness: A Brief History*, Oxford: Oxford University Press

Porter, R. (2006) *Madmen: A Social History of Madhouses, Mad-Doctors and Lunatics*, Stroud, Glos.: Tempus Publishing Ltd

Prentky, R.A. (2001) 'Mental illness and roots of genius', *Creativity Research Journal*, 13(1): 95–104

Preti, A. and Miotto, P. (1997) *Creativity, Evolution and Mental Illnesses*. Available at: http://cfpm.org/jom-emit/1997/vol1/preti_a&miotto_p.html (accessed March 2014)

Prinzhorn, H. (1922) *Artistry of the Mentally Ill: A Contribution to the Psychology and Psychopathology of Configuration*, E. von Brockdorff (trans.), 2nd German edn, reprint New York, Heidelberg, Berlin: Springer-Verlag

Putland, C. (2008) 'Lost in translation: the question of evidence linking community based arts and health promotion', *Journal of Health Psychology*, 13: 265–276

Quality Care Commission (2010) 'Count me in', Results of the 2010 national census of inpatients and patients on supervised community treatment in mental health and learning disability services in England and Wales. Available at: www.cqc.org.uk/sites/default/files/media/documents/count_me_in_2010_final_tagged.pdf (accessed March 2014)

Repper, J. and Perkins, R. (2003) *Social Inclusion and Recovery*, Edinburgh: Balliere Tindall

Rexer, L. (2005) *How to Look at Outsider Art*, New York: Harry N. Abrams

Rhodes, C. (2000) *Outsider Art: Spontaneous Alternatives*, London: Thames and Hudson

Richards, R., Kinney, D.K., Lunde, I., Benet, M. and Merzel, A.P. (1988) 'Creativity in manic-depressives, cyclothymes, their normal relatives, and control subjects', *Journal of Abnormal Psychology*, 97: 281–288

Richardson, F.C. and Guignon, C.B. (2008) 'Positive psychology and philosophy of social science', *Theory and Psychology*, 18(5): 605–627

Ricoeur, P. (1970) *Freud and Philosophy: An Essay on Interpretation*, Binghamton, NY: Yale University Press

Ricoeur, P. (1986) 'Life: a story in search of a narrator', in M. Doeser and J. Kray (eds) *Facts and Values*, Dordrecht: Martinus Nijhoff

Ricoeur, P. (2012) *On Psychoanalysis*, Cambridge: Polity Press

Riessman, C. (2002) 'Analysis of personal narratives', in J.F. Gubrium and J.A. Holstein (eds) (2000) *Handbook of Interview Research: Context and Method*, London: Sage Publications, 695–710

Rilling, J., Gutman, D., Zeh, T., Pagnoni, G., Berns, G. and Kilts, C. (2002) 'A neural basis for social cooperation', *Neuron*, 35(2): 395–405

Roberts, G.A. (2000) 'Narrative and severe mental illness: what place do stories have in an evidence-based world?' *Advances in Psychiatric Treatment*, 6(6): 432–441

Roberts, J. (2007) *The Intangibilities of Form*, London: Verso Books

Rosenhan, D.L. (1973) 'On being sane in insane places', *Science*, 179: 25–28

Rothenberg, A. (1990) *Creativity and Madness: New Findings and Old Stereotypes*, Baltimore: Johns Hopkins University Press

Royal College of Psychiatrists (2010) 'No health without public mental health: the case for action', Position statement: Available at: www.rcpsych.ac.uk/pdf/Position%20 Statement%204%20website.pdf (accessed March 2013)

Rush, B. (1812) *Medical Inquiries and Observations upon the Diseases of the Mind*, Philadelphia, PA: Kimber & Richardson

Rustin, M. (2001) *Reason and Unreason: Psychoanalysis, Science and Politics*, London: Continuum International

Sagan, O. (2007a) 'Research with rawness: the remembering and repeating of auto/ biographical ethnographic research processes', *Ethnography and Education*, 2(3): 349–364

Sagan, O. (2007b) 'An interplay of learning, creativity and narrative biography in a mental health setting: Bertie's story', *Journal of Social Work Practice*, 21(3): 311–321; and also in P. Chamberlayne (ed.) *Art, Creativity and Imagination in Social Work Practice*, London: Routledge, 4: 53–63

Sagan, O. (2009a) 'Anxious provision and discourses of certainty: the sutured subject of mentally ill adult learners', *International Journal of Lifelong Education*, 28(5): 615–629

Sagan, O. (2009b) 'Uninterrupted: mentally ill students' narratives of learning and creating', *International Journal of Interdisciplinary Social Sciences*, 4(8): 203–212

Sagan, O. (2012) 'Continua – mentally ill artist students uninterrupted', in A. Bainbridge and L. West (eds) *Psychoanalysis and Education: Minding a Gap*, London: Karnac Books, 5: 177–197

Sagan, O. (2013) 'Stories my father never told me', in E.D. Miller (ed.) *Stories of Complicated Grief: A Critical Anthology*, Washington, DC: NASW Press, 15: 255–267

Santosa, C.M., Strong, C.M., Nowakowska, C., Wang, P.W., Rennicke, C.M. and Ketter, T.A. (2007) 'Enhanced creativity in bipolar disorder patients: a controlled study', *Journal of Affective Disorders*, 100(1–3): 31–39

Sarbin, T.R. (ed.) (1986) *Narrative Psychology: The Storied Nature of Human Conduct*, New York: Praeger Publications Inc.

Sass, L.A. (2001) 'Schizophrenia, modernism, and the "creative imagination": on creativity and psychopathology', *Creativity Research Journal*, 13(1): 55–74

Sawyer, R.K. (2006) *Explaining Creativity: The Science of Human Innovation*, New York: Oxford University Press

Scharfstein, B. (2009) *Art without Borders: A Philosophical Exploration of Art and Humanity*, Chicago: University of Chicago Press

Schaverien, J. (1993) 'The retrospective review of pictures: data for research in art therapy', in H. Payne (ed.) *Handbook of Inquiry in the Arts Therapies: One River, Many Currents*, London: Jessica Kingsley

Scheff, T.J. (1999) *Being Mentally Ill*, 3rd edn, New York: Aldine de Gruyter

Schiff, A.C. (2004) 'Recovery and mental illness: analysis and personal reflections', *Psychiatric Rehabilitation Journal*, 27(3): 212–218

Schildkraut, J.J., Hirschfeld, A.J. and Murphy, J.M. (1996) 'Depressive disorders, spirituality and early deaths in the abstract expressionist artists of the New York School', in J.J. Schildkraut and A. Otero (eds) *Depression and the Spiritual in Modern Art*, Chichester: John Wiley & Sons

Schlesinger, J. (2002) 'Issues in creativity and madness part one: ancient questions, modern answers', *Ethical Human Sciences and Services*, 4(1): 73–76

Schlesinger, J. (2009) 'Creative myth conceptions: a closer look at the evidence for the "mad genius" hypothesis', *Psychology of Aesthetics, Creativity, and the Arts*, 3(2): 62–72

Schreber, D.P. [1903] (2000) *Memoirs of My Nervous Illness*, New York: New York Review Books Classics

Schuldberg, D. (2001) 'Six subclinical spectrum traits in normal creativity', *Creativity Research Journal*, 13(1): 5–16

Scull, A. (1984) *Decarceration: Community Treatment and the Deviant – a Radical View*, 2nd edn, London: Basil Blackwell

Secker, J., Hacking, S., Spandler, H., Kent, L. and Shenton, J. (2007) *Mental Health, Social Inclusion and the Arts: Developing the Evidence Base*, London: National Social Inclusion Programme, Care Service Improvement Partnership

Secker, J., Hacking, S., Kent, L., Shenton, J. and Spandler, H. (2009) 'Development of a measure of social inclusion for arts and mental health project participants', *Journal of Mental Health*, 18(1): 65–72

Segal, H. (1974) 'Delusion and artistic creativity: some reflections on reading *The Spire* by William Golding', *International Journal of Psychoanalysis*, 1: 135–141

Segal, J. (1992) *Melanie Klein*, London: Sage Publications

Self, A. and Randall, C. (2013) *Measuring National Wellbeing – Review of Domains and Measures*, Office for National Statistics. Available at: http://ons.gov.uk/ons/dcp171766_308821.pdf (accessed March 2014)

Seligman, M.E.P. and Csikszentmihalyi, M. (2000) 'Positive psychology: an introduction', *American Psychologist*, Millennial Issue 55(1): 5–15

Seneca (c. 4 BC–CE 65), Epistles

Sennett, R. (2012) *Together: The Rituals, Pleasures and Politics of Cooperation*, London: Allen Lane

Shenton, M., Dickey, C., Frumin, M. and McCarley, R. (2001) 'A review of MRI findings in schizophrenia', *Schizophrenia Research*, 49(1): 1–52

Shriver, L. (2010) *So Much for That*, London: Harper

Simeonova, D.I., Chang, K.D., Strong, C. and Ketter, T.A. (2005) 'Creativity in familial bipolar disorder', *Journal of Psychiatric Research*, 39: 623–631

Simonton, D.K. (2010) 'So you want to become a creative genius? You must be crazy!' in D.H. Cropley, A.J. Cropley, J.C. Kaufman and M.A. Runco (eds) *The Dark Side of Creativity*, Cambridge, MA: Cambridge University Press, 12: 218–234

Smith, E.R., Murphy, J. and Coats, S. (1999) 'Attachment to groups: theory and measurement', *Journal of Personality and Social Psychology*, 77: 94–110

Spandler, H., Secker, J. and Kent, L. (2007) 'Catching life: the contribution of arts initiatives to recovery approaches in mental health', *Journal of Psychiatric and Mental Health Nursing*, 14(8): 791–799

Spiegelberg, H. (1982) *The Phenomenological Movement: A Historical Introduction*, 3rd edn (with the collaboration of Karl Schuhmann), The Hague: Marinus Nijhoff

Spitz, E.H. (1989) *Art and Psyche: Study in Psychoanalysis and Aesthetics*, New Haven: Yale University Press

Stacey, G. and Stickley, T. (2010) 'The meaning of art to people who use mental health services', *Perspectives in Public Health*, 130(2): 70–77

Stern, D. (1985) *The Interpersonal World of the Infant*, New York: Basic Books

Stickley, T. (2010) 'Does prescribing participation in arts help to promote recovery for mental health clients?' *Nursing Times*, 106(18): 18–20

Stickley, T. (ed.) (2012) *Qualitative Research in Arts and Mental Health*, Ross-on-Wye: PCCS Books

Stickley, T., Hui, A., Morgan, J. and Bertram, G. (2007) 'Experiences and constructions of art: a narrative discourse analysis', *Journal of Psychiatric and Mental Health Nursing*, 14: 783–790

Stokes, A. (1965) *The Invitation in Art*, New York: Chilmark Press Inc.

Stone, B. (2004) 'How can I speak of madness? Narrative and identity in memoirs of "mental illness"', in *Narrative, Memory and Identity: Theoretical and Methodological Issues*, Huddersfield: University of Huddersfield, 49–57

Stone, B. (2006) 'Diaries, self-talk, and psychosis: writing as a place to live', *Auto/Biography*, 14: 41–58

Storr, A. (1993) *The Dynamics of Creation*, New York: Ballantine Books

Strong, C.M., Nowakowska, C., Santosa, C.M., Wang, P.W., Kraemer, H.C. and Ketter, T.A. (2007) 'Temperament-creativity relationships in mood disorder patients, healthy controls and highly creative individuals', *Journal of Affective Disorders*, 100(1–3): 41–48

Szasz, T. (1960) 'The myth of mental illness', *American Psychologist*, 15: 113–118

Szasz, T. (1974) *The Myth of Mental Illness*, London: Paladin

Tagore, R. (2002) *Stray Birds*, New Delhi: Rupa & Co.

Teall, W., Tortora-Cailey, A. and Cunningham, J. (2006) *Voyage on a Painted Sea: A Life in a Day*, Brighton: Pavilion Journals, 10: 7–11

Thomson, M. (1989) *On Art and Therapy*, London: Virago

Townsend, P. (2013) 'Making space', in A. Kuhn (ed.) *Little Madnesses: Winnicott, Transitional Phenomena and Culture Experiences*, New York: I.B. Tauris, 14: 173–187

Tusa, J. (1999) *Art Matters: Reflecting on Culture*, London: Methuen

Vellante, M., Zucca, G., Preti, A., Sisti, D., Rocchi, M.B.L., Akiskal, K.K. and Akiskal, H.S. (2011) 'Creativity and affective temperaments in non-clinical professional artists: an empirical psychometric investigation', *Journal of Affective Disorders*, 135: 28–36

Waddell, C. (1998) 'Creativity and mental illness: is there a link? Review Paper', *Canadian Journal of Psychiatry*, 43(2): 166–172

Wadlington, W. and McWhinnie, H.J. (1973) 'The development of a rating scale for the study of formal aesthetic qualities in the paintings of mental patients', *Art Psychotherapy*, 1: 201–220

Wahl, O.F. (1995) *Media Madness: Public Images of Mental Illness*, Piscataway, NJ: Rutgers University Press

Wallin, D.J. and Johnson, S. (2007) *Attachment in Psychotherapy*, Guildford: Guildford Publications

Walsh, M. (2013) *Art and Psychoanalysis*, London: I.B. Tauris

Wengraf, T. (2001) *Qualitative Research Interviewing: Biographic Narrative Semi-Structured Methods*, London: Sage Publications

White, M. (2005) *Genning Up: A Research Paper for Blue Drum on Community-Based Arts in Health*, CAHHM, University of Durham

White, M. (2006) 'Establishing common ground in community-based arts in health', *Journal of the Royal Society of Health*, 126(3): 128–133

White, M. (2009) *Arts Development in Community Health: A Social Tonic*, Abingdon: Radcliffe

White, M. (2010) in P. Devlin, 'Restoring the balance: the effect of arts participation on wellbeing and health'. Available at: www.voluntaryarts.org/wp-content/uploads/2011/10/Restoring-the-Balance.pdf (accessed March 2014)

White, M. (2011) 'Arts in Health – a new prognosis', IXIA website article available at: www.ixia-info.com (accessed March 2014)

Wigram, T. and Gold, C. (2012) 'The religion of evidence-based practice: helpful or harmful to health and wellbeing?' in R. MacDonald *et al.* (eds) *Music, Health and Wellbeing*, Oxford: Oxford University Press, 164–182

Winnicott, D.W. (1953) 'Transitional objects and transitional phenomena', *International Journal of Psychoanalysis*, 34: 89–97

Winnicott, D.W. (1971) *Playing and Reality*, New York: Pelican Books, 1985

Winnicott, D.W. (1991) *Playing and Reality*, London: Routledge

Wood, D. (1991) *On Paul Ricoeur: Narrative and Interpretation*, London: Routledge

World Health Organization (2002) *Gender Disparities in Mental Health*. Available at: www.who.int/mental_health/prevention/genderwomen/en/ (accessed June 2014)

Wright, K. (2009) *Mirroring and Attunement: Self-Realization in Psychoanalysis and Art*, London: Routledge

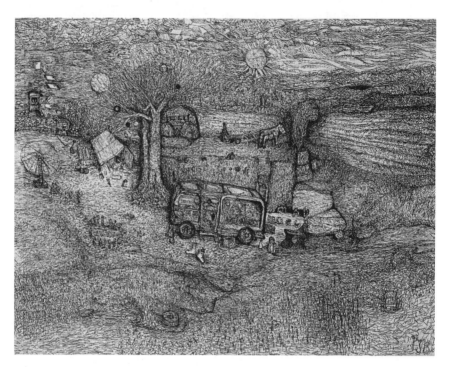

Bring your own television

Index

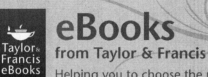

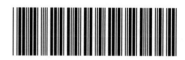